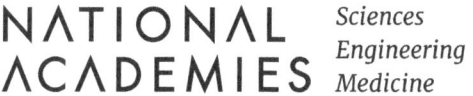
NATIONAL ACADEMIES PRESS
Washington, DC

Community Interventions to Prevent Veteran Suicide

The Role of Social Determinants

Laura Yoder, *Rapporteur*

Board on Behavioral, Cognitive, and Sensory Sciences

Division of Behavioral and Social Sciences and Education

Proceedings of a Virtual Symposium

THE NATIONAL ACADEMIES PRESS 500 Fifth Street, NW Washington, DC 20001

This activity was supported by a contract between the National Academy of Sciences and the U.S. Department of Veterans Affairs (36C24518D0171/36C24521N0414). Any opinions, findings, conclusions, or recommendations expressed in this publication do not necessarily reflect the views of any organization or agency that provided support for the project.

International Standard Book Number–13: 978-0-309-69102-4
International Standard Book Number–10: 0-309-69102-8
Digital Object Identifier: https://doi.org/10.17226/26638

This publication is available from the National Academies Press, 500 Fifth Street, NW, Keck 360, Washington, DC 20001; (800) 624-6242 or (202) 334-3313; http://www.nap.edu.

Copyright 2022 by the National Academy of Sciences. National Academies of Sciences, Engineering, and Medicine and National Academies Press and the graphical logos for each are all trademarks of the National Academy of Sciences. All rights reserved.

Printed in the United States of America.

Suggested citation: National Academies of Sciences, Engineering, and Medicine. (2022). *Community Interventions to Prevent Veteran Suicide: The Role of Social Determinants: Proceedings of a Virtual Symposium.* Washington, DC: The National Academies Press. https://doi.org/10.17226/26638.

The **National Academy of Sciences** was established in 1863 by an Act of Congress, signed by President Lincoln, as a private, nongovernmental institution to advise the nation on issues related to science and technology. Members are elected by their peers for outstanding contributions to research. Dr. Marcia McNutt is president.

The **National Academy of Engineering** was established in 1964 under the charter of the National Academy of Sciences to bring the practices of engineering to advising the nation. Members are elected by their peers for extraordinary contributions to engineering. Dr. John L. Anderson is president.

The **National Academy of Medicine** (formerly the Institute of Medicine) was established in 1970 under the charter of the National Academy of Sciences to advise the nation on medical and health issues. Members are elected by their peers for distinguished contributions to medicine and health. Dr. Victor J. Dzau is president.

The three Academies work together as the **National Academies of Sciences, Engineering, and Medicine** to provide independent, objective analysis and advice to the nation and conduct other activities to solve complex problems and inform public policy decisions. The National Academies also encourage education and research, recognize outstanding contributions to knowledge, and increase public understanding in matters of science, engineering, and medicine.

Learn more about the National Academies of Sciences, Engineering, and Medicine at **www.nationalacademies.org**.

Consensus Study Reports published by the National Academies of Sciences, Engineering, and Medicine document the evidence-based consensus on the study's statement of task by an authoring committee of experts. Reports typically include findings, conclusions, and recommendations based on information gathered by the committee and the committee's deliberations. Each report has been subjected to a rigorous and independent peer-review process and it represents the position of the National Academies on the statement of task.

Proceedings published by the National Academies of Sciences, Engineering, and Medicine chronicle the presentations and discussions at a workshop, symposium, or other event convened by the National Academies. The statements and opinions contained in proceedings are those of the participants and are not endorsed by other participants, the planning committee, or the National Academies.

Rapid Expert Consultations published by the National Academies of Sciences, Engineering, and Medicine are authored by subject-matter experts on narrowly focused topics that can be supported by a body of evidence. The discussions contained in rapid expert consultations are considered those of the authors and do not contain policy recommendations. Rapid expert consultations are reviewed by the institution before release.

For information about other products and activities of the National Academies, please visit www.nationalacademies.org/about/whatwedo.

**PLANNING COMMITTEE ON COMMUNITY
INTERVENTIONS TO PREVENT VETERAN SUICIDE:
THE ROLE OF SOCIAL DETERMINANTS**

TIMOTHY J. STRAUMAN (*Chair*), Duke University
LISA A. BRENNER, University of Colorado
MITZI A. FIELDS, U.S. Army
DEBRA HOURY, Centers for Disease Control and Prevention
EVELYN L. LEWIS, Veterans Health and Wellness Foundation
RAJEEV RAMCHAND, RAND Corporation

MOLLY CHECKSFIELD DORRIES, *Study Director*
JEANNE RIVARD, *Senior Program Officer*
ASHTON BULLOCK, *Senior Program Assistant*

BOARD ON BEHAVIORAL, COGNITIVE, AND SENSORY SCIENCES

TERRIE E. MOFFITT (NAM) (*Chair*), Duke University
RICHARD N. ASLIN (NAS), Yale University
JOHN BAUGH, Washington University in St. Louis
WILSON S. GEISLER (NAS), The University of Texas at Austin
MICHELE GELFAND (NAS), University of Maryland, College Park
ULRICH MAYR, University of Oregon
KATHERINE L. MILKMAN, University of Pennsylvania
ELIZABETH A. PHELPS, Harvard University
DAVID E. POEPPEL, New York University
STACEY SINCLAIR, Princeton University
TIMOTHY J. STRAUMAN, Duke University

SAMANTHA CHAO, *Acting Director*

Acknowledgments

This Proceedings of a Virtual Symposium was reviewed in draft form by individuals chosen for their diverse perspectives and technical expertise. The purpose of this independent review is to provide candid and critical comments that will assist the National Academies of Sciences, Engineering, and Medicine in making each published proceedings as sound as possible and to ensure that it meets the institutional standards for quality, objectivity, evidence, and responsiveness to the charge. The review comments and draft manuscript remain confidential to protect the integrity of the process.

We thank the following individual for their review of this proceedings: Evelyn L. Lewis, Veterans Health and Wellness Foundation, Rutgers Robert Wood Johnson Medical School. We also thank staff member Tracy Lustig for reading and providing helpful comments on this manuscript.

Although the reviewers listed above provided many constructive comments and suggestions, they were not asked to endorse the content of the proceedings nor did they see the final draft before its release. The review of this proceedings was overseen by Bernadette M. Melnyk, Vice President for Health Promotion and University Chief Wellness Officer, and Dean, College of Nursing, The Ohio State University. She was responsible for making certain that an independent examination of this proceedings was carried out in accordance with standards of the National Academies and that all review comments were carefully considered. Responsibility for the final content rests entirely with the rapporteur and the National Academies.

Contents

1 INTRODUCTION   1
Structure of Symposium and Proceedings, 2

2 SOCIAL, CULTURAL, AND ECONOMIC DETERMINANTS
RELATED TO SUICIDE, PANEL 1   5
Financial Wellbeing as a Social Determinant of Suicide Risk
   in Veterans, 6
Setting the Stage: The Significance of Social Determinants of
   Health, 8
Overview of Trends in Suicide in *High and Rising Mortality
   Rates Among Working-Age Adults*, 11
Discussion, 13

3 SOCIAL, CULTURAL, AND ECONOMIC DETERMINANTS
RELATED TO SUICIDE, PANEL 2   15
Veterans in Rural Areas, 15
Native American/Alaska Native Veterans, 19
Women Veterans, 23
Discussion, 26

4 SOCIAL, CULTURAL, AND ECONOMIC DETERMINANTS
RELATED TO SUICIDE, PANEL 3   29
LGBTQ+ Veterans, 30
Black American Men and Provider Role Strain, 33
Discussion, 36

5	COMMUNITY INTERVENTIONS FOR SUICIDE PREVENTION AND SUPPORT FOR VETERANS	39

Upstream Prevention by Addressing Social Determinants of Health, 40
Community-Driven Efforts to Prevent Firearm Suicide, 42
The CDC Technical Package on Suicide Prevention, 45
Discussion, 48

6	COMMUNITY INTERVENTIONS FOR VARIED APPLICATIONS IN HOUSING, HEALTH, AND SAFETY	51

Housing and Homelessness, 51
Using a Collaborative Approach in Suicide Prevention, 53
Place-Based Interventions, 55
Discussion, 58

7	REPORTS FROM INTERACTIVE SESSION GROUPS	59

Older Veterans, 60
LGBTQ+ Veterans, 60
Veterans in Rural Communities, 61
Mental Health, 62
Black Veterans, 63
Women Veterans, 64

8	DISCUSSION OF INTERACTIVE SESSION REPORTS AND SYNTHESIS OF THE SYMPOSIUM	67

Cross-Cutting Themes Across Interactive Sessions, 68
Synthesis of the Symposium, 71

REFERENCES	73

APPENDIXES
A	Symposium Agenda	77
B	Biographical Sketches of Planning Committee Members and Presenters	83

1

Introduction

On March 28 and 29, 2022, the Board on Behavioral, Cognitive, and Sensory Sciences at the National Academies of Sciences, Engineering, and Medicine held a virtual symposium entitled *Community Interventions to Prevent Veteran Suicide: The Role of Social Determinants*, which was the product of a collaboration begun in June 2020 between the U.S. Department of Veterans Affairs (VA) and the National Academies aimed to address "social, cultural, and economic factors influencing suicide risk among veterans, and to in turn identify best practices for suicide prevention, intervention, and postvention at the community level," said Matthew Miller (Department of Veterans Affairs Suicide Prevention Program). He went on to explain that the symposium's focus on the social determinants of health as they relate to veteran suicide prevention was built around three central tenets adopted by Miller's team at the VA. The first of these tenets is that suicide is preventable. The second tenet is that suicide prevention will require a public health approach wherein challenges are addressed via policies, procedures, and programs that address the needs of the entire population as well as those at highest risk; promote equitable distribution and access to clinical care and support; and address the role of social and ecological risk and prevention factors. The third tenet highlights the importance of each participant's contribution in the work of suicide prevention. Miller expressed hope that the symposium would "inspire and invigorate each of us regarding the meaningful and unique roles every one of us and each of us can play."

In his overview of the symposium agenda, planning committee chair Timothy Strauman (Duke University) highlighted the two central goals

> **BOX 1-1**
> **Statement of Task**
>
> The National Academies of Sciences, Engineering, and Medicine will appoint a planning committee to organize an open, two-day virtual symposium to gain a better understanding of social determinants influencing the recent increase in suicide risk and how currently available practice guidelines can inform community-level preventive interventions, particularly those targeting veteran populations. The symposium will address: (1) the relevant social, cultural, and economic factors driving changes in suicide risk among veterans and (2) ways that current best practices for suicide prevention and treatment can be applied at the community level.
>
> A rapporteur will prepare a proceedings to summarize the discussion at the symposium and be reviewed in accordance of institutional guidelines.

articulated in the Statement of Task: to gain a clearer picture of the social determinants that might move veterans toward distress and suicide risk, and to identify existing best practices for suicide prevention and treatment used in community-based interventions that could be employed to help reduce suicide risk in veterans in particular. Strauman noted that the identification of new opportunities for prevention would also be part of the agenda, with the goal of generating "new ideas that are doable, exciting, and inspiring," a process meant to "help jumpstart what we think is a new chapter in preventing suicide for veterans," said Strauman. (See Box 1-1 for Statement of Task.)

STRUCTURE OF SYMPOSIUM AND PROCEEDINGS

The symposium took place virtually over two days. The first day featured a combination of presentations, panel discussions, and question and answer sessions as participants "hear[d] from experts on the social, cultural, and economic determinants of suicide risk, particularly among veterans, as well as from experts who are engaged in community-based preventive interventions that are targeting those determinants," according to Strauman. The second day saw participants divided into groups to discuss community prevention as it relates to a specific population of veterans; a reporting session and discussion where each breakout group shared their work with the larger group; and finally, a synthesis of the symposium sessions by the Planning Committee. This proceedings follows the structure of the symposium. Chapters 2 through 6 cover the presentations made over the course of the first day of the symposium. The following chapters cover the second day, with summaries of the reports from each breakout group in Chapters 7 and large-group discussion of this material in Chapter 8. Chapter 8 also includes the synthesis generated in the final session of the symposium.

This proceedings has been prepared by the symposium rapporteur as a factual summary of what occurred at the symposium. The planning committee's role was limited to planning and convening the symposium. The views contained in the proceedings are those of individual symposium participants and do not necessarily represent the views of all symposium participants, the planning committee, or the National Academies of Sciences, Engineering, and Medicine.

2

Social, Cultural, and Economic Determinants Related to Suicide, Panel 1

The first panel of speakers was introduced by moderator Debra Houry, who noted that the session's overview of the evidence on social, cultural and economic determinants of suicide "will help us form the basis for much of what we're doing." Houry continued, "During today's session our panels will share some of the risk and protective factors for suicide, and the factors related to suicide among the general population and veterans, as well as the implications for preventing suicide through interventions." The panel included three panelists: Eric Elbogen (Duke University) presented on financial factors as significant social determinants of health, including risk of suicide morbidity (i.e., suicidal ideation, suicide attempt, and mortality linked with suicide); Sandro Galea (Boston University School of Public Health) provided an overview of social determinants of health and how they might be used in developing more effective interventions; and Irma Elo (University of Pennsylvania) provided an overview of trends in suicide mortality in the report *High and Rising Mortality Rates Among Working-Age Adults* (NASEM, 2021).

FINANCIAL WELLBEING AS A SOCIAL DETERMINANT OF SUICIDE RISK IN VETERANS

> *Financial problems significantly increase the odds of suicidal ideation and suicide attempts, Elbogen stated. His presentation shows how improving financial wellbeing of veterans through financial education and connecting them with financial resources and tools can provide an upstream approach that can ultimately help to prevent and reduce risk of suicide.*

Elbogen began his discussion of financial wellbeing as one of multiple factors that form social determinants of health in relation to suicide risk among veterans by emphasizing the financial challenges that service members face at the point of separation from the military, often, becoming financially independent for the first time at a later age than their civilian counterparts. Veterans are more likely to incur debt and be delinquent on debt payments, he noted. Elbogen continued, these financial struggles occur alongside challenges in employability that veterans encounter as they transition out of the service; these might include the need to retrain to transfer work skills to the civilian sector, and physical and mental health injuries that might affect employability.

Such challenges are consequential, contributing to financial wellbeing as a social determinant of risk for suicide morbidity, Elbogen said. He cited a study whose "an extensive analysis [of VA medical records] confirmed that for veterans . . ., financial problems increased odds of suicidal ideation and suicide attempts significantly, even controlling for other risk factors" (Blosnich et al., 2019). This mirrors the link between financial strain and suicide evident in the general population, he noted (Richardson et al., 2013).

Elbogen stressed that financial wellbeing "doesn't occur in a vacuum" but is part of a constellation of risk and protective factors. He pointed to findings in the National Post-Deployment Adjustment Survey (2020), a survey he led which investigated whether protective factors, including financial wellbeing, predicted suicidal ideation. The survey looked at eight psychosocial protective factors, some of which related to financial wellbeing, like employment and having money for basic needs. The study found having more of these eight psychosocial protective factors, including financial wellbeing, was associated with a significant drop in suicidal ideation one year later (from 60% for those having zero protective factors to 3% for those having all eight protective factors), Elbogen reported.

This was similar to findings within the general population, Elbogen said. His team looked at the National Epidemiologic Survey on Alcohol and Related Conditions (NESARC), a survey of more than 34,000 people in the United States, conducted by the National Institutes of Health. This dataset showed that individuals with financial debt and crisis, a history of homelessness, and a history of unemployment, and were below median income were 20 times more likely to attempt suicide in the next three years compared with those who did not have any financial risk factors, Elbogen said. "The cumulative financial strain was significant even when controlling for depression, substance use, and history of suicide attempts and ideation." Examination of this same NESARC dataset using machine learning by researchers at Columbia University identified the top 20 predictors of suicide attempts out of the 2,500 variables included in the dataset (de la Garza et al., 2021), said Elbogen. He observed that within the top 20 predictors, 4 had to do with financial strain, "showing that there is a link between financial strain and suicide risk" in the general population.

Elbogen then turned to financial strategies and money management interventions that have been used to address financial strain that, as a result, have the potential to decrease the risk of suicide. He cited a meta-analysis of 29 studies that showed that financial strategies do have a medium effect size in terms of reducing spending and increasing saving (Davydenko et al., 2021). Elbogen noted that this and other research shows the importance of establishing a specific reason for financial goals: "I'm saving up for X because I value Y." This includes techniques like using technology to create an avatar of the user as an older person to concretize the idea of saving for the future, he said. $teps for Achieving Financial Empowerment ($AFE) is an intervention program developed by Elbogen and his team, funded by the Department of Education, to help veterans learn strategies that promote financial wellbeing. $AFE uses this same strategy of associating a financial goal with a psychosocial SMART goal. Elbogen emphasized that the importance here lies in the fact that these psychosocial goals add a sense of self-determination. He briefly listed other ways to help relieve financial strain for veterans, including helping veterans attain work, avoid scams, and access veteran-specific discounts (including awareness of a page on the VA website that lists available discounts).

Elbogen closed his presentation by reiterating that financial stability is one of many protective factors, and that "developing financial stability and other psychosocial protective factors can be viewed especially from the lens of social determinants of suicide as a critical part of community success." He noted that things service members have when they are in the military—including stable housing, a job, social support, basic needs met, a sense of mission—may no longer be present when they transition into civilian life. Supporting the financial wellbeing of veterans (by connecting them to financial tools, financial resources, and financial education) "can provide an upstream approach to ultimately help prevent and reduce risk of suicide."

SETTING THE STAGE:
THE SIGNIFICANCE OF SOCIAL DETERMINANTS OF HEALTH

> *Addressing/mitigating risks of social determinants of health among veterans in addition to biomedical factors would yield more effective interventions, and yet the United States devotes significantly less funding to research in this domain compared to biomedical solutions. This leads to "sicker and shorter lives" in the U.S, said Galea. He advocates for addressing public health solutions through a framework that includes social determinants of health. Within the veteran population, he said, primary social factors that determine risk of suicide ideation or suicide attempt are (1) life course (not just isolated events); (2) social supports; (3) mental health; and (4) ubiquity of challenges.*

More attention needs to be paid to social determinants of health because they contribute "substantially more to health than does health care and medicine," said Galea in his overview of the social determinants of health. He noted that in terms of the "production of health," "health care is maybe 10 to 20 percent of health" while "most of our health actually comes from" socioeconomic factors, physical environment, and health behaviors (i.e., social determinants of health). However, in the United States, funding and support are focused primarily on health care, resulting in a mismatch between health determinants and health expenditures, with 90 percent of national health expenditures devoted to health care services and 9 percent to healthy behaviors, Galea said. This in turn results in "sicker and shorter lives," where the United States lagged behind other countries in life expectancy (Roser, 2017). He called out the importance of this symposium's focus on social determinants of health within the "array of factors that are relevant."

Galea illustrated the importance of attending to social determinants of health by recounting the life of Blind Willie Johnson, a blues musician from Texas, born at the turn of the 20th century. Galea described a host of injuries and challenges Johnson encountered over the course of his life before dying at age 40 of malaria, after having been denied care when taken to a hospital. Galea observes that "it's very clear that it wasn't just malaria that killed Blind Willie Johnson;" social determinants of health—including domestic violence, homelessness, poverty, racism, poor access to health care—played a significant role. Focusing only on the prevention and treatment of malaria would not have given him a "healthier, longer life," Galea argued, and noted that similarly, in the United States today, focusing medicine and treatment alone will not lead to "longer, healthier lives. Ultimately, the social determinants are a nondiscretionary part of the determinants of health," Galea summarized.

Galea presented a conceptual framework for thinking about "a full set of social determinants of health" and how different level forces interact with and influence one another (see Figure 2-1). Using this framework, Galea discussed four points about social determinants of health as they relate to suicide risk and prevention for veterans. The first point is that social determinants manifest over the life course. "We tend to think of veterans' health or military health as indexed to military experience, and we tend to forget that the military experience actually is part of a full continuum of lifetime experiences." To illustrate this, Galea pointed to a study that connected onset of depression with adverse childhood events within a National Guard cohort; though assessment might focus on military experiences, in fact "it is adverse events during childhood that matter" in this case.

Galea's second point is that social support can be a protective factor in maintaining health in general. This can be seen in a study that looked at factors associated with deployment-related posttraumatic stress; this study

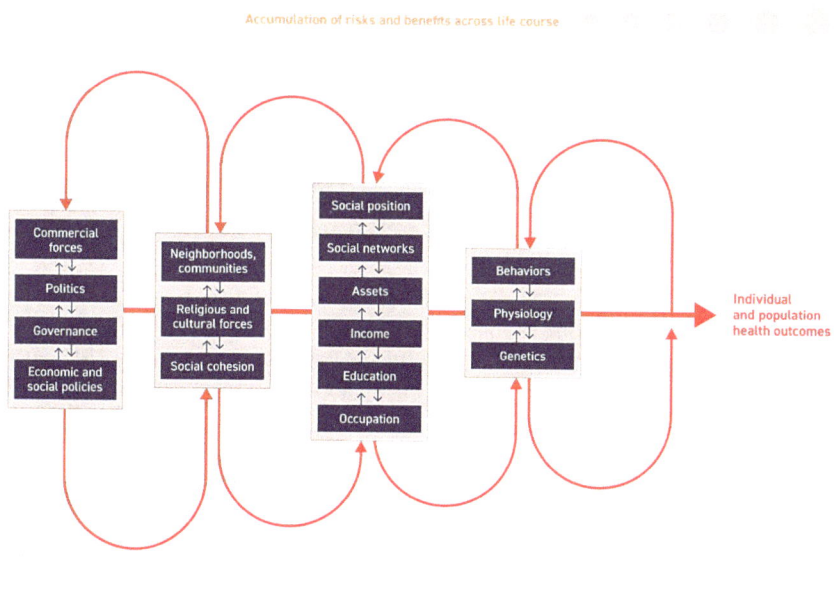

FIGURE 2-1 Social determinants, life course, and health.
SOURCE: *Data, Social Determinants, and Better Decision-Making for Health: The Report of the 3-D Commission* (2021), presentation by Galea (slide 13).

found an association between low levels of preparedness and support with high prevalence of posttraumatic stress disorder (PTSD). Galea also pointed to a study showing that low social support "is substantially associated with greater risk of suicidal ideation."

The third of these four points Galea makes is that when investigating the social determinants of suicide, one must also attend to the determinants of other mental health disorders that are themselves determinants of risk—that is, "the full range of mental health factors that are coincident with, and some antecedent to, suicidal ideation." For example, one study shows that those with PTSD are four times more likely to report suicidality than those without, said Galea, while those with PTSD and two or more other disorders are eight times more likely to report suicidality than those without.

Galea's fourth and final point had to do with "ubiquity" which he defined as "forces that are present everywhere." Ubiquity, he said, describes social determinants that are "all around us" and sometimes, because of this, "very hard to think of them." He gave the example of loneliness and isolation as contributing factors in the increase in drug overdose deaths in the past year. Ubiquity describes "something that has deep impact that we actually don't think about," he explained.

Galea closed with a reiteration of the importance of social determinants and the problems with basing public health solutions primarily on medical treatments. He illustrated this through a brief recounting of an ongoing argument about the causes of starvation among children that unfolded between two public health advocates in 19th-century England, Edwin Chadwick and William Farr. Farr showed that poverty was a significant contributor to childhood death in England; Chadwick focused on micronutrient deficiency as the cause of death. Galea noted that both are right, but that interventions centered primarily on correcting a micronutrient deficiency would not actually address the problem in a complete way. Similarly, "we as a society tend to privilege thinking about and talking about our biomedical approach, a pillable approach, and tend to underprivilege conversation about all these other forces." Noting that this is not an "either/or argument" between a biomedical approach and engagement with social determinants, Galea urged the development of "comprehensive approaches" that bring to bear "this full range of determinants."

PANEL 1

OVERVIEW OF TRENDS IN SUICIDE IN *HIGH AND RISING MORTALITY RATES AMONG WORKING-AGE ADULTS*

> *The 2021 report* High and Rising Mortality Rates Among Working-Age Adults *examines social determinants of health as part of what is driving the recent increase in mortality rates among middle-aged Americans, said Elo. Looking at upstream factors as well as proximate determinants of health, and at the entire life course, the authoring committee found that explanations for this increase centered on four main factors: mental and emotional health; economic wellbeing; social engagement, religious participation, and social support; and access to lethal means, she said.*

Elo presented findings on trends in suicide mortality in *High and Rising Mortality Rates Among Working-Age Adults* (NASEM, 2021), a consensus study report by the National Academies of Sciences, Engineering, and Medicine, in the third panel of this session. This study was guided by a framework of social determinants of health and provides insight into increasing mortality rates among middle-aged Americans, "particularly from causes referred to as "deaths of despair" that included suicide, alcohol-related causes, and drug overdose." While it did not focus on veterans' suicide, many of the factors visible in this big-picture view pertain to veterans as well, Elo said.

The study was designed to investigate possible causes behind "big increases" in mortality rates and a decline in U.S. life expectancy from 2014 to 2018, Elo explained. She set the stage by reviewing these data, which show that deaths from substance abuse and mental health (including drug poisoning, alcohol-induced death, mental and behavioral causes, and suicide) "were the main reasons" for decline in U.S. life expectancy during this time. Changes in mortality as seen in standardized death rates between 1990 and 2017 show widespread increases across three age groups spanning 25 to 64: non-Hispanic White males, non-Hispanic Black males, and Hispanic males; data for females is similar. Elo called out the particularly big increase in death by drug poisoning, which included suicide by drug poisoning, for women ages 25–44. Turning to suicide mortality particularly, she noted that rates increased in almost all states with some variation across the country, particularly for ages 25–65, and especially in rural areas.

Elo said that the committee's approach to analysis relied on a "comprehensive framework" of social determinants of health. This included attending to upstream factors (e.g., social, political, and cultural contexts that included such things as federal, state, and local policies; corporate and business practices; social and economic inequality; and culture) and "meso-level structural factors" (e.g., family context, social networks, work environments, health care, physical and built environment), and their effects on individual and proximate determinants of health. The committee similarly took a big-picture approach in considering experiences and factors across the life course, including early life.

Elo reports that the committee found that explanations for suicide centered on four factors:

1. Mental and emotional health
2. Economic factors
3. Social engagement, religious participation, and social support
4. Access to lethal means

Elo elaborated briefly on each of these areas. She noted that in the area of mental and emotional health, the committee "witnessed [a] rise in hopelessness, stress, and poor mental health," including an increase in stressful life events, in the United States during this period of time. She listed other factors that increase individuals' risk of suicide, including psychiatric disorders, impulsivity, prior suicide attempts, and family history of suicide. These factors also interact with broader cultural, social, and economic contexts, she noted.

Of economic factors, Elo said, "very few studies looked at causal processes; however, there is ample evidence that there is a strong association between economic disruptions, financial strain, and suicide." Within this area, she said, the committee identified factors related to employment, such as loss of manufacturing and mining jobs in rural areas and wage stagnation or decline, as well as housing foreclosure rates and changes to social safety net programs. Many of these factors had a stronger association with individuals with lower levels of schooling, she said.

Trends in various forms of social engagement, religious participation, and social support were also offered as possible explanations for rising suicide rates during the period of study, Elo said. These included loss of social networks concomitant with job loss, a decline in civic participation, decreases in religious affiliation and church attendance, and, at the family level, increasing divorce rates and increases in single-parent families. In general, "much of the social and cultural trends have diminished access to social support" that would be a protective factor against suicide.

Access to lethal means is a major factor in suicide rates, said Elo. She noted the strong association between firearm availability and suicide rates, pointing to data that show that states with looser gun regulations also tend to have higher firearm-related rates of suicide. Firearm-related suicides are much higher in rural areas, and more prevalent among men, she continued. Elo also noted increases in the use of other modalities that contribute to the overall increase in rates of suicide. These include higher rates for suicide by drug poisoning, especially by women.

Elo closed her presentation by mentioning that data from 2019 and 2020 "suggest suicide mortality has not increased during the pandemic, perhaps contrary to our expectations."

DISCUSSION

The discussion began with a question from committee member Rajeev Ramchand, who brought up the interplay between financial stress and mental health and, within that, the role of mental health workers in helping veterans navigate financial stressors as part of mental health care. Elbogen noted that psychologists might be involved "to the extent that financial stressors begin to interact with mental health problems." But he emphasized the importance of knowing the limits of psychological treatment and making referrals to financial experts in cases where the area of need extends beyond the realm of mental health.

Strauman noted the huge range of social determinants mentioned in the three presentations and wondered about raising awareness around the fact that there is such a big range of factors and broadening the general understanding of what these many factors are. He added that if the "word already is out," what could be done to help systematize and support this message. Galea responded by emphasizing how difficult it can be to communicate about that health "inextricable" from socially determined factors, but that the present social movements and social context may be a turning point, with "disgust" about racial and economic inequities around COVID-19 acting as a catalyst for including social determinants in conversations about health. It is, he argued, "our collective responsibility" to include social determinants in discussions about health so as to create "political pressure . . . to act on the social determinants." Elo concurred, remarking "I do think that a lot of it depends on political will to do something about it." She voiced some skepticism over whether recent attention to social determinants of health "will translate into real action given the biomedical community's bigger presence in the political discussions," but noted that "I think it does take all of us to make that happen." And she reiterated the statement that "until social determinants of health are better addressed, the United States continues to fall behind" in life expectancy. Elbogen referenced fundamental attribution errors (i.e., focusing on individual characteristics at the expense of broader contextual determinants) as one possible reason for the tendency to ignore social determinants. Evelyn Lewis added that awareness around the importance of social determinants—in all their various forms—has been raised again and again over the years in piecemeal ways that rarely impact "upstream" issues such as medical training; she remarked that this perspective needs to be "integrated into the full spectrum of what [medical personnel, all members of the medical team] needs to be considered during their patient interactions" if any lasting downstream results are to be expected. Galea reinforced this, noting, "in the broader conversation, we keep thinking that if we just act good enough downstream, it's going to be good enough." Blosnich pointed to the importance of social workers within the medical infrastructure as those trained in connecting people to resources.

Subsequent discussion points included the existence of financial education offered to veterans by the military through the Office of Financial Readiness; the research potential of a question that asks, are there "sets of social circumstances," including adverse child experiences, that then contribute to putting people in harm's way—that is, making them "more at risk for other adverse social circumstances," said Galea; and the importance of support, connectedness, and belonging in combatting adverse circumstances but also—with the creation of an in-group, or clique—exacerbating them. The final point of discussion Houry raised for this panel was the future of veteran suicide prevention. Galea emphasized bridging the VA and community efforts, and making sure that veterans return to supportive community. Elbogen emphasized the interrelationship of protective factors, and pointed to the importance of encouraging "that underlying sense of self determination, control, and hope in the future." Elo mentioned the potential of targeted interventions for individuals; such interventions would be built on knowledge of specific risk factors associated with a higher risk of suicide.

Strauman closed the panel by pointing to the potential of interdisciplinary collaboration; "extending suicide prevention to include (from an academic perspective) disciplines like sociology, anthropology, nursing, economics" has the potential to "include a really broad base of community stakeholders."

3

Social, Cultural, and Economic Determinants Related to Suicide, Panel 2

Evelyn Lewis moderated the second panel of the virtual first session, which focused on special populations within the veteran population. Nathanial Mohatt (Department of Veterans Affairs) reviewed some of the evidence on rural social determinants of health and risk factors that are related to suicide both in the general population and among veterans in particular. Pamela End of Horn (Indian Health Service [IHS] Headquarters) discussed morbidity and mortality of American Indian and Alaska Native (Native) populations and how that is correlated to native veterans. Claire Hoffmire (Department of Veterans Affairs, University of Colorado School of Medicine) addressed social determinants of health and risk factors as related to suicide rates among women veterans.

VETERANS IN RURAL AREAS

A variety of factors more prevalent in rural communities than in urban ones may be contributing to much higher rates of suicide in the former, Mohatt said. These factors include poverty, poor access to health care, and geographic isolation.

Rates of suicide are much higher in rural communities of the United States than in urban ones, Nathaniel Mohatt told the group. As a rule, the rural classification includes a range from any town with 50,000 people or fewer to open, empty spaces. He explained that rural in the United States includes 97 percent of U.S. land, 18 percent of the population, and 24 percent of veterans specifically. There is also a great deal of diversity to be found in these rural areas, Mohatt said. Rural communities are not only diverse in terms of population density, but areas with economic, cultural, and educational diversity. While rural economies were historically primarily agricultural, with 40 percent of jobs in that sector 100 years ago, at present less than 1 percent of rural jobs are in agriculture and rural economies are more reliant on other sectors like "retail, tourism and outdoor recreation, health care, and education," said Mohatt. Culturally, rural areas are often thought of as being primarily White; while there is a higher proportion of White people living in rural communities than in urban ones, he noted, cultural diversity is growing, particularly in the Hispanic/Latinx community. Mohatt also noted a general assumption that people in rural communities have less education than their urban counterparts; while people in rural areas do "on the whole have lower educational attainment," this does not mean that "rural people are uneducated or unaware of what's going on in the world, or unable to think deeply about life."

Mohatt then discussed three factors within the social determinants of health in rural areas that account for at least some of the disparity between rural and urban suicide rates: poverty, poor access to health care, and geographic isolation. Of poverty, he noted that not only do rural areas have relatively high poverty rates, but also, a higher proportion of rural counties are at the worst level of deprivation compared with urban counties. Access to health care is another challenging area; 65 percent of rural counties are designated as health care workforce shortage areas, with very few specialty providers. This means that people living in rural areas are less likely to receive needed treatment for mental health and substance use. As such, rural residents "have a higher disease burden," explained Mohatt, "so the mental illness that they're experiencing . . . lead[s] to greater burden or greater problems from the same levels of diagnoses that exist in urban areas." Finally, he noted, geographic isolation in rural communities can lead to greater social isolation, which disproportionately impacts vulnerable populations. One such population is older adults who can no longer drive; similarly, people with disabilities and people with mental illness challenges can "become increasingly more socially isolated."

Suicide rates are increasing more quickly in rural areas than urban communities, Mohatt said, and "this disparity has been widening over the past 30 years." Rural veterans have a 14 percent to 20 percent increased risk of death by suicide compared with urban veterans, he said. Mohatt noted that breaking this number down by race and ethnicity reveals several reasons for the disparity between rural and urban rates of suicide. The first is that "growth in suicide among Hispanic Americans in rural communities has grown faster" than rates of suicide for Hispanic Americans in urban areas. This disparity between urban and rural areas is not evident in data on rates of suicide among Black and White populations, Mohatt observed. The second reason for the higher rates of suicide in rural areas seen when breaking data down by race and ethnicity is that there are more rural White veterans than urban White veterans, proportional to other races. Non-Hispanic Whites and non-Hispanic Natives had the "highest suicide rates across all three urbanization levels, with both groups experiencing greater increases compared with non-Hispanic blacks, non-Hispanic Asian/Pacific Islanders, and Hispanics across the study period" (Ivey-Stephenson et al., 2017). The third is that a much higher proportion of Native American veterans live in rural areas than urban communities, compared with other races, and this population is the highest risk racial group with the highest suicide rates. These trends all contribute to the disparity between rural and urban rates of suicide among veterans: higher proportions of White and Native American veterans, and a faster rate among rural Hispanic veterans.

Mohatt noted that while understanding risks for suicide among rural White populations is an important part of "understanding rural suicide in the United States," attributing higher suicide rates in rural America to a proportionately higher White population in those areas is oversimplifying the problem and "doesn't help us understand why there are higher suicide rates in rural places where there aren't White Americans with guns." Rates of suicide are higher in rural communities not just in the United States but internationally; international literature can help identify factors beyond race that contribute to this disparity between rural and urban suicide rates, he said. Factors cited by international literature on rural rates of suicide include geographic isolation and lack of access to services—in themselves factors as discussed above—which can contribute to cultural factors like stigma toward mental illness, stoicism, and self-reliance. Economic factors include the impact of natural disasters on agricultural areas and the impacts of economic downturn on the farming sector. Environmental factors include lethal means, said Mohatt; while firearms are used more frequently in rural communities than in urban areas in the United States, international data show high rates of suicide by poisoning from pesticides. Social isolation is an interpersonal factor, while chronic health disparities and mental health disease burden also are shown in international literature to play a significant role, he said.

A systematic review conducted by Mohatt et al. (2020) of data show several factors for the rural/urban disparity within the United States that particularly impact Native American communities, he said. First, the disparity in suicide rates "among rural adults is largely driven by lethal means," he said; "if you control for firearms, that rural/urban disparity either goes completely away or mostly goes away." Second, data point to substance use, particularly alcohol, as a comorbidity with suicide attempts and suicide deaths in rural communities, with higher prevalence among men and in Native American populations. Third, Mohatt noted that there are not a lot of data linking poor access to health care and higher rates of suicide, but that the literature does show a "persistent disparity" between urban and rural communities in this area, particularly mental health care. This will "continue to be a barrier to our ability to do suicide prevention if you don't figure out either creative ways around [this lack] or new ways to get better access to mental health care in rural communities," said Mohatt. Fourth, he noted that the review found that financial and economic factors do not contribute *more* to suicide risk in rural communities than in urban ones, and so do not explain the disparity between the two; but they do *contribute* to rural suicide.

In addition to these factors that increase risk of suicide, Mohatt noted, rural areas also possess strengths that can possibly be leveraged to decrease risk of suicide. These include the land itself as a source of peace and quiet as well as recreation and shared pursuits; a culture of resilience; social capital (i.e., "people are fewer degrees separated from decision makers in rural communities in general"); and, a culture of self-reliance which, at the community level, is a culture of collective agency—coming together to overcome adversity.

Mohatt et al. (2020) found a lack of studies around the impact of "community-level factors like access to care and financial risk" on suicide rates in rural communities, Mohatt said. "There are fewer studies, and lower evidence quality." He continued, "in terms of suicide prevention, most best practices haven't been examined relative to rural needs." He emphasized the need for further research and work into questions of "how do we design our services and our programs to better meet the needs of rural areas."

As one example of how community-based suicide prevention efforts might be used for rural veterans in particular, Mohatt pointed to the VA's Together With Veterans (TWV) program. This program is veteran-driven, collaborative, evidence-based, and community-centered; in collaboration with rural communities, this becomes about collaborating with rural communities to draw on their strengths—particularly in the area of social capital—to establish more effective prevention interventions, he said. This includes "training rural veterans to become public health leaders in their communities." Such training can serve as a "force extender to the health care community that is resource-strapped," Mohatt said. Training laypeople to be public health planners has been shown to be effective in this program, he noted.

NATIVE AMERICAN/ALASKA NATIVE VETERANS

> *Recent data show that suicide rates among American Indian and Alaska Native populations, including veterans, already disproportionately high, are increasing, End of Horn said. She reviewed two promising strategies for addressing this problem: community-based outreach that connects Native veterans with VA resources as well as IHS resources; and including traditional healers in clinical settings.*

End of Horn's presentation focused on the social determinants of health, and suicide as alongside other health outcomes, among Native populations. She began by describing social determinants that affect the population as a whole and then turned to how these factors particularly impact the Native veteran population.

Native people comprise about 1.7 percent of the U.S. population, with 574 tribes recognized by the federal government as sovereign nations, and more than 300 different languages, End of Horn said. She described several features of this population: they are a "mobile population," with many moving between reservations and urban areas, sometimes with two homes and sometimes without a fixed home and living with family. This group is also multicultural—different nations, bands, and families comprise this group, End of Horn noted.

Natives serve at the highest rate of any minority in the military, with members from all tribes, End of Horn said. This makes for about 150,000 currently serving, with women making up 10 percent of that number. Native service members are "very different from their compatriots in other races," she continued. These differences include a tendency to live in the west; a lower median age (59 years as opposed to 64 years of other races); lower personal income; more likely to lack health insurance; and more likely to have a service-related disability.

Native service members are also impacted by factors that affect the entire population, End of Horn continued. These include a lower life expectancy (78 years compared with 80 years for the non-Hispanic White population); high disease burden; inadequate education; disproportionate rates of poverty and economic adversity; difficulty starting and maintaining a business under federal jurisdiction (i.e., on a reservation); discrimination and racism; and poor social conditions, including gang violence and other crime. End of Horn also noted that Native veterans also face a lack of access to local, county, and state services. Because of living on a federal reservation or trust land, they may only have access to tribal services or the IHS, she said.

End of Horn observed that because of these challenges, Natives are often thought about or approached by others via a "perspective of deficiency." This perception of deficiency contrasts with the high esteem and respect afforded to veterans within the community, and, together, these conflicting elements can prompt Natives to join the military, End of Horn suggested. Natives leave the reservation and community to better themselves—to overcome this perceived deficiency—and to emulate family members who may be veterans highly respected within the community. She noted that often veterans then return to their home communities and that "often [these veterans are] one of the more core groups on the reservation that are willing to do a lot more for specifically elderly and for children."

The mortality rates among Natives are an important factor in understanding the situation for Native veterans in particular, End of Horn said. The average age of death is 78 years old, which is lower than the non-Hispanic White population; additionally, "they are suffering from a high rate of morbidity," she noted. Pointing to data from the IHS, she noted that heart disease, cancer, diabetes, and unintentional injuries/accidents are more prevalent among the Native population than the general U.S. population. The first three can result from "historic inadequacies" of food, with a lack of access to "green leafy vegetables" and a diet heavy in processed carbohydrates a contributing factor to the particularly high rates of diabetes. The high mortality rate associated with accidents is associated with living and working in rural areas, often on a farm or ranch with livestock, End of Horn noted. She also pointed to the especially high rate of mortality due to of alcohol abuse and related health conditions, as well as the high rates of infectious disease such as influenza, pneumonia, and now, COVID-19 (see Figure 3-1).

Suicide was the eighth leading cause of death across all ages among Native populations in 2017, making up 18 percent of total deaths (640 of 3,447). End of Horn reported. This is a higher rate of suicide than other races and ethnic groups, she noted. Of these suicide deaths, 46.6 percent were by suffocation/hanging and 38.6 percent were by firearms; End of Horn said that "depending on what dataset you look at," firearms are sometimes shown to be more prevalent than suffocation, "but the reality is, it's both."

One of the most difficult parts of suicide prevention in Native communities is stigma, End of Horn said. "Suicide as a word is very taboo in a lot of our tribal communities," who believe that in saying the word, "we're bringing it into awareness." This results in a stigma around suicide that can be a barrier for struggling individuals who might not seek needed mental health services because of this cultural pressure.

American Indian/Alaska Native Population and Mortality Rates[3]

INDIAN HEALTH SERVICE

	AI/AN Rates 2009-2011	U.S. All Rates Rate – 2010	Ratio AI/AN to U.S. All Races
All Causes	999.1	747.0	1.3
Diseases of the heart (Heart Disease)	194.7	179.1	1.1
Malignant neoplasm (cancer)	178.4	172.8	1.0
Accidents (unintentional injuries)*	93.7	38.0	2.5
Diabetes mellitus (diabetes)	66.0	20.8	3.2
Alcohol-induced	50.0	7.6	6.6
Chronic lower respiratory diseases	46.6	42.2	1.1
Cerebrovascular diseases (stroke)	43.6	39.1	1.1
Chronic liver disease and cirrhosis	42.9	9.4	4.6
Influenza and pneumonia	26.6	15.1	1.8
Drug-induced	23.4	15.3	1.5

FIGURE 3-1 American Indian/Alaska Native population and mortality rates.
SOURCE: Presentation by End of Horn (slide 5).

Not a lot is known about Native veterans as a group, because most of the data come from two health care systems—the VA and the IHS—that approach care and data tracking from two different perspectives, said End of Horn. The VA attends to individuals as veterans, while the IHS data reflect individuals' identity within the Native population, she said. In addition to this difference in perspective, the two systems also have different ways of taking in data, which makes it difficult to identify and begin to understand this population, End of Horn observed.

Among Native veterans, the suicide rate has more than doubled, with ages 18–39 having the highest rate, End of Horn reported (Mohatt et al., 2022). She noted that this highest risk for suicide among younger veterans reflects the higher risk of young people within the larger Native population. Additionally, risk of suicidal ideation is twice as high for Native veterans as for non-Hispanic White veterans, she said.

End of Horn concluded her presentation with a discussion of some strategies for meeting the needs of Native veterans. She advocated for community-based outreach done via building relationships through networking, "meaning finding an individual, getting them connected, and then having them make connections for you," rather than cold calling or other non-relationship-based forms of outreach. This would involve getting to know individuals and finding out what their specific needs are, she noted.

Another effective strategy was the inclusion of traditional healers and traditional practices, End of Horn said. She cited the inclusion of a traditional healer in the Veterans Integrated Service Networks (VISN23) of the VA at the St. Paul VA Medical Center in St. Paul, Minnesota, as a contributor to good outcomes at that institution. "The traditional healer within the community often bridged the gap for Native veterans to get into services and result in actually coming and getting care." End of Horn emphasized that in this situation, participation *in traditional practices* often served to connect Native veterans with the VA. She noted that the IHS often includes traditional practices as an element of care and includes healers on the care team, if desired by the patient.

Finally, End of Horn pointed to the complex interplay of two health care systems—the VA and the IHS—and noted that many Native veterans get care through IHS but eschew the VA. Bridging this gap and helping Native veterans take advantage of available services in the VA is an important area of inquiry, she suggested. She noted the importance of having VA staff, including social workers, who are able to help resolve issues that come up when learning a new system. Having "peer support providers who are Native veterans who can help other Native veterans . . . would be the most beneficial to Native veterans overall." This is because Native peer support providers might be able to bridge cultural barriers, she said. Additionally, "chances are, they're going to trust that [peer] more so than anybody else simply because that Native person may understand the system a lot better, is working in the system, and able to provide information in a way that would really connect them" to these services in a way that will truly help not just achieve a specific goal and get relevant services but, ultimately, "help [Native veterans] increase their quality of life." Native veterans are so important to traditional communities and beliefs, End of Horn said, that "serving Native veterans is one of the highest things we can do."

WOMEN VETERANS

> *Social determinants of health can impact men and women differently, and gender itself is a social determinant of health, Hoffmire explained. Addressing suicide risk for women veterans should involve looking at and addressing social determinants of health as they particularly impact women. These include housing and financial concerns; justice involvement; homelessness; barriers to health care access; and military sexual trauma.*

Hoffmire's presentation focused on how social determinants of health impact women veterans in particular. She began by reminding listeners that gender itself is a social determinant of health; additionally, "we should expect that other social determinants of health impact outcomes differentially by gender as well." She sketched an overview of women in the military, women veterans, and suicide rates compared with male veterans. Following this, Hoffmire discussed three studies that showed fluctuations in the risk for suicide and instances of suicidal ideation over the life course. She then reviewed some of the factors that impact rates of suicidal morbidity in women veterans. And finally, Hoffmire considered the close connection between wellbeing and social determinants in light of separation from the military for women veterans and suicide risk in that population.

About 10 percent of veterans are women; this is one of the fastest growing subgroups of veterans, and projected to reach approximately 16–17 percent around 2043, said Hoffmire. As in the general population, the rate of suicide for female veterans is lower than for male veterans. Hoffmire pointed to data showing that, for Western cultures, "across the vast majority of populations, females have higher rates of suicidal ideation and non-fatal suicidal behavior, but lower rates of suicide" when compared to males. The comparative rates of suicide among female and male veterans reflect this, Hoffmire noted. She continued, 2001 to 2017 saw a "substantial" increase in rates among women veterans. From 2017–2019, there was "a pretty notable decline in suicide rates among our female veterans;" while this decline is "promising," it is not clear if it is a long-term trend, she said.

Data show that the risk of suicide differs at different points within the life course of the female veteran, Hoffmire said. "The relationship between suicide rates and time since leaving military service appears to differ for men and women, but considering overall rates when evaluating such trends may mask variable trajectories of risk over the period of reintegration into civilian life. Understanding drivers of high-risk trajectories is critical." Hoffmire pointed to one study on veteran suicide rates by sex and time since separation that showed that for male veterans, the suicide rate is highest at the point of separation and then decreases over the next seven years (Bullman et al., 2015). This same study showed that for women, there did not seem to be a decrease in risk for suicide. Data on suicidal ideation after separation from the military over a three-year integration period, gathered by Hoffmire and colleagues, does not show meaningful gender differences, she reported (Hoffmire et al., 2022). There may, however, be differences in predictors of suicidal ideation trajectories post-separation from military service, she said.

Hoffmire pointed to a third study, this one focused on women veterans, that showed "a high lifetime rate of suicidal ideation, attempt, and nonsuicidal self-injury, with prevalence of both ideation and attempt higher following separation from service than the women experienced prior to and during military service" (Monteith et al., 2020). However the onset of suicidal morbidity (i.e., "the time that women veterans indicate they first experienced ideation and attempt") among this group was most often pre-military, Hoffmire reported. Thus many women veterans have some prior ideation or attempt that already puts them at risk, she said.

Another study by Hoffmire and colleagues compares women veterans to non-veteran women, non-veteran men, and to male veterans, she said. "In comparison to non-veteran women, we found that women veterans experienced a higher prevalence of ideation and attempt in adulthood but not in childhood and adolescence," she reported (Hoffmire et al., 2021). Additionally, for women veterans, the odds of ideation and attempt onset were increased in adulthood relative to childhood, while for non-veteran women, the odds were decreased in adulthood.

Turning to a consideration of the social determinants of suicide risk for women veterans, Hoffmire summarized, "We know that gender is clearly a determinate of suicide risk among our veterans." For women in particular, she noted that data are scarce but "increasingly available." Hoffmire stated, "delineating specific factors, including social determinants of health, driving suicide risk for women veterans, overall and at specific times across the life course, is essential." She said that one growing area of research is psychosocial stressors and differences of their impact by gender. Hoffmire briefly reviewed such stressors, including the following:

- Housing and financial concerns. Hoffmire noted that, in one study, housing and financial concerns associated with suicidal ideation among female veterans but not male veterans, "whereas concerns about other recent stressful life events were associated with ideation only among males."
- Justice involvement. Hoffmire reported that another study found that female justice-involved veterans were three times more likely

to report a lifetime suicide attempt than women veterans without a history of justice involvement. She also noted that most research in this area has been focused on male veterans, but recent data show this as an important social determinant for women veterans.
- Homelessness and housing instability. Women veterans who have experienced homelessness and housing instability have been shown to be at "even greater risk for suicide attempts," Hoffmire explained.
- Access as a barrier to health care. In 2017 and 2018, the age-adjusted suicide rate for non–Veterans Health Administration (VHA) female veterans exceeded that of VHA female Veterans. However, the majority of women veterans do not use VHA services and women encounter unique barriers to health care access, she continued. For example, 25 percent of women veterans report experiencing harassment at VHA health care centers, which "may result in delayed or missed care," Hoffmire reported. Challenges around childcare also disproportionately affects women veterans seeking care. Finally, a historic lack of gender-sensitive care within VHA has also presented challenges for women as well as any veteran seeking care related to gender identity; though substantial efforts have and continue to be to provide more care of this kind, she noted.
- Military sexual trauma (MST) and interpersonal violence. Hoffmire reported that women who have a history of MST often have a lower willingness to use VHA if they're suicidal or experiencing mental health challenges. This aversion might be the result of many factors, Hoffmire noted, citing "institutional betrayal" as one possibility.

"Certainly we can address suicide risk for our women veterans by looking at and addressing social determinants of health" including these psychosocial stressors as they particularly impact women, Hoffmire summarized.

One growing area of research around the mitigation of these psychosocial stressors and the decrease of suicide risk is through a framework of the concept of wellbeing, Hoffmire said. Wellbeing includes an individual's health (physical and mental) as well as vocational, financial, and social circumstances, with the latter three considered aspects of psychosocial wellbeing, she noted. Hoffmire said that these aspects of psychosocial wellbeing overlap greatly with social determinants of health—and that social determinants of health greatly contribute to psychosocial wellbeing; but, she explained, the two are distinct in that social determinants of health "typically focus on status" while psychosocial wellbeing is concerned with "functioning and satisfaction" in addition to status. For example, in the area of finances, income is a social determinant of health whereas financial wellbeing also includes a person's sense of satisfaction and how they are functioning within various financial domains.

Hoffmire pointed to the Wellbeing Inventory (WBI) (Vogt et al., 2019), a multidimensional assessment tool developed with veteran populations to measure status, functioning, and satisfaction within four life domains: health, vocation (work and education), finances, and social relationships (intimate, community, parenting). She reported that data gathered as part of the Veterans Metrics Initiative Study (in progress) on overall wellbeing show an association of higher levels of wellbeing with a lower likelihood of "high-risk trajectories of ideation" among both male and female veterans. A second study using the WBI focused on women veterans using VHA reproductive health care services shows that in the domain of parenting, there is "a threefold increase in the prevalence of current [suicidal] ideation among women who reported low versus high satisfaction in their parenting," reported Hoffmire (in progress). Status (whether or not someone is a parent) and functioning, however, were not associated with suicidal ideation. These findings point to "the importance of continuing to study the intersection between parenting and suicide risk among women veterans," she noted. Hoffmire concluded her presentation by gesturing to several ongoing studies that will expand knowledge regarding social determinants of suicide risk for women veterans, including consideration of the impact that COVID-19 might have on the risk for suicide among this population.

DISCUSSION

Discussion for this panel was moderated by Lewis and began with a consideration of the impact of an increase in rural populations due to relocation from urban centers spurred by the COVID-19 pandemic. Mohatt expressed worry that the health system in rural areas is "already overextended, overtaxed." This is the result of "negative trends in access to care over the last five years plus," including difficulty attracting providers to rural areas and hospital closures "because the economics of rural health care are just really challenging." He did note that one thing to hope for is that an increase in population will bring with it an increase in money within the local economy and so help mitigate some of the deficits.

Hoffmire addressed the need for intersectional research that attends to the experiences of women veterans of color, and the question of why current studies are not designed to include subpopulations from the start. She noted that while this is an important area of research, feasibility is a problem in that women veterans are already a small minority subgroup, and getting a big enough sample can be difficult; "most studies don't have enough women veterans to make meaningful informative conclusions about women veterans as a whole," let alone subgroups. Two ways of correcting this limitation in future studies would be to design studies that address specific subpopulation questions or to design large-scale studies that oversample women and veterans of color to yield enough data to analyze different subgroups and do comparative analysis, Hoffmire said. She noted the present importance of the second type of study as a way of identifying factors that are particularly important for certain subgroups that might then receive more focused study.

End of Horn discussed why some of the strategies for reducing suicide risk mentioned in her presentation have not been implemented in a robust way within the VA and the IHS health care systems. She reiterated the importance of having representation within the VA system, not just for Native populations but for other religious affiliations. She also noted that Native veterans come to the IHS over the VA in part because "we're right there" on the reservation, making access easier. End of Horn suggested the importance of "getting outside of the medical center . . . and going to the community," leveraging connections and presence within a community to slowly connect and built trust with Native veteran representatives, not just tribal leaders.

Discussing the problems of racism and discrimination as they appear in rural areas, Mohatt pointed to an in-progress survey of all veterans participating in TWV, a rural suicide prevention program. Preliminary findings show the training topic of most interest to study participants is "diversity, equity, and inclusion," he reported. There is "a very strong interest in learning more about diversity and culture as it relates to suicide, and how to be more engaged across cultures and communities in rural areas."

The final part of the discussion concerned the further development of connections between large agencies such as the VA and veteran-owned, veteran-run small organizations around prevention of veteran suicide. Mohatt pointed to the TWV program as one example of the VA doing this: "it's completely built and predicated on the idea of engaging with rural veterans and rural veterans' service organizations to ensure that veterans are the leaders of community-based suicide prevention." Hoffmire spoke to the importance of involving veteran partners from various subgroups in order to make sure that studies include their perspective throughout the process, from design to data gathering to the dissemination of results.

4

Social, Cultural, and Economic Determinants Related to Suicide, Panel 3

The third and final panel in the session on social, cultural, and economic determinants related to suicide was moderated by Rajeev Ramchand and featured presentations on two groups within the general veteran population: sexual and gender minority populations, and Black/African American men. John Blosnich (University of Southern California and the Center for Health Equity Research and Promotion at the Pittsburgh VA) described some of the disparities in suicide risk and prevention among lesbian, gay, bisexual, and transgender individuals as seen through the lens of social determinants of health. Sean Joe (Washington University in St. Louis) spoke on the social determinants of suicide that impact Black American men, focusing in particular on factors that contribute to "provider role strain" that, in turn, can be a factor for suicide risk. Like the other panelists in this second session, Blosnich and Joe look at how data about specific populations might interact with research done on suicide prevention more generally and "introduce a slight detour in those conversations," as Blosnich put it.

LGBTQ+ VETERANS

> *LGBTQ+ veterans have a higher prevalence of suicide morbidity than the general veteran population, said Blosnich. Strategies for preventing suicide should be informed by recent evidence that shows that social determinants of health can affect this population differently. Additionally, LGBTQ+ identity is not represented in administrative datasets of mortality rates, which leads makes it difficult, if not impossible, to measure mortality and disease burden for this subpopulation, which in turn makes it difficult to establish outcomes and direct resources.*

Blosnich presented on sexual and gender minority (SGM) populations within the veteran population, focusing on the health equity implications for LGBTQ+ people as seen in suicide prevention. He opened his presentation by highlighting some common terms of gender identity, pointing to the United States Transgender Survey, which shows many "evolving terms" related to gender identity in the United States. He stressed that gender identity is distinct from sexual orientation, which includes self-identification, sexual attractions, and sexual behavior; and that gender identity does not depend on medical interventions or medical therapies. Citing data from the Behavior Risk Factor Surveillance System (BRFSS) (2016) conducted by the Centers for Disease Control and Prevention (CDC), Blosnich noted that many people who identified their gender identity as transgender identified their sexual orientation as heterosexual. He also observed that the BRFSS introduced an optional module for sexual orientation and gender identity in 2014, which allows for probability-based samples rather than convenience-based samples that were (and are) more common in research about LBGT populations. Blosnich noted that a 2021 Gallup survey found that 5.6 percent of Americans identify as LGBT, and found that it is much more common for people in younger generations to identify as LGBT than those in older generations (Jones, 2021).

Blosnich noted that research on suicidal ideation and attempt consistently shows much higher rates among sexual and gender minority populations than those of the general population or their cisgender and heterosexual counterparts. He noted that these disparities for these sexual minorities can be seen in one meta-analysis of studies conducted by Hottes et al. (2016), *Lifetime Prevalence of Suicide Attempts Among Sexual Minority Adults by Study Sampling Strategies: A Systematic Review and Meta-Analysis*. This review found that 4 percent of people identified as heterosexual had considered or attempted suicide over their lifetime, compared with 17 percent of people identified as a sexual minority. Blosnich also mentioned his own scoping review of reviews from 1990–2022, of 32 review studies that covered 1,148 studies, all of which supported the finding that "the prevalence of suicide morbidity is much higher" in this population.

Blosnich then turned to suicide research among sexual and gender minority veterans. He noted that doing research on this population is challenging because self-identified sexual orientation and gender identity data are currently "not represented in administrative data" at the VA. In a 2021 study, Boyer et al. using VA records had to "mine through data to find indicators that would suggest that a patient was a sexual minority." In a different study about transgender veterans, they used *International Classification of Diseases* (ICD) coding to help identify a subset of veterans "who we would think are transgender." This study revealed that while suicide was the tenth leading cause of death for cisgender veterans in the United States, it was the fourth for transgender veterans. Similarly, the rate of suicide was the fifth leading cause of death for LGB veterans, compared with the tenth leading cause for non-LGB veterans and also the U.S. population. Blosnich noted that these sampled were "probably underestimated."

Blosnich then considered some specific social determinants that might explain these disparities in the rates of suicide morbidity. He pointed to the concept of minority stress found in the work of Virginia Brooks and further developed by Ilan Meyer as a way of understanding how stigma drives health disparities experienced by sexual and gender minority people. Blosnich noted that this model is predicated on distal and proximal stressors. The former, he explained, includes processes outside the person, including structural discrimination, laws, and policies. The latter describes intra-personal conditions, of, for example, "someone . . . internalizing the stigma that is leveled against them by society." All of these features of minority stress impact the mental and physical health of the individual, Blosnich said. They also produce societal strains that lead to adverse social determinants, he noted. Blosnich pointed to two examples of how stigma drives social determinants, found in the VA study of transgender veterans. There, a universal screen for MST and housing instability showed that transgender veterans are "much more likely" to screen positive for both MST and housing instability compared with their cisgender peers. Similarly, Blosnich reported that data from the BRFSS show a high prevalence of nearly all adverse childhood experiences in the LGB population.

Blosnich then briefly gestured to research that seeks to quantify how larger societal elements like policies and legislation can become associated with mental and physical health outcomes for sexual and gender minority populations, including studies that show how "social environmental factors supportive of sexual and gender minorities have protective associations against suicide ideation [and] attempt." He also pointed to family determinants (i.e., how supportive the family is) as a risk or protective factor that might differ for LGBT populations. For that group, Blosnich commented, the family might be a source of rejection and distress rather than support; conversely, he noted, a study by Russell et al. (2018) shows that one indicator associated with lower depressive symptoms and lower prevalence of suicidal ideation and suicidal attempt for a transgender young person is the family's acceptance and use of a chosen name that affirms the child's gender identity.

Blosnich then elaborated on two examples where traditional suicide prevention interventions might be reconsidered in light of data showing how social determinants might affect LGBTQ+ veterans differently than the general veteran population or civilian population. These areas are religion/religiosity and firearms. Blosnich noted that the National Strategy for Suicide Prevention emphasizes faith-based partnerships, based on research that having a religious identity is usually a protective factor against suicide. He reported that his own study of 20,000 young adults and the importance of religious or spiritual beliefs to personal identity shows this, revealing that among people who identify as heterosexual, those who said religion was important to them had lower odds of reporting suicide ideation. For bisexual participants, there were no significant associations between religiosity and suicidal ideation, but for lesbian, gay, or questioning participants, there was an opposite association; those in that population who said they were more religious were more likely to say they had suicidal ideation in the past year. He observed that this difference "challenges us to think about how we can work with faith-based partners to make sure that a health equity lens is brought to suicide prevention" and, more broadly, to make sure that *all* partners in the work of suicide prevention are helping to understand where these disparities are coming from.

The second example Blosnich gave in using data to rethink traditional prevention approaches is firearms as a determinant for death by suicide. He reports that BRFSS data from California and Texas reveals that in both states, "sexual minorities are significantly less likely to report having a firearm in their household compared to their heterosexual peers." While these communities had high prevalence in other known risk factors for suicide (including previous attempts, previously thinking about suicide, and actively thinking about suicide), the lower prevalence of this particular determinant was "a good sign," Blosnich observed, and wondered if "less access to firearms could be a protective feature that we just do not really fully understand yet in this population." Access to firearms is still a significant factor in suicide deaths for transgender veterans, he continued, but less so for this group than for the cisgender veteran population. At the same time, the rate of suicide death by poisoning is much higher for transgender veterans than their cisgender peers. Blosnich observes that these differences should, again, prompt reflection about how prevention interventions affect specific subgroups as well as the entire population. "If we devote a lot of resources into gun safety, which is important for all populations, is it still going to have as big an effect for this sample, transgender veterans, as opposed to looking into more prevention for death by self-poisoning, for example?"

Blosnich closed his presentation by discussing the absence of mortality data for LGBT people. This lack of representation in administrative datasets means that research showing that LGBT people are more likely to have risk factors for suicide but cannot be connected to mortality outcomes to determine if rates of suicide death are elevated. He observes, "We cannot get to these ultimate outcomes and that absolutely puts the brakes on prevention because we cannot adequately measure the burdens of disease." Because of this, too, he notes, resources cannot be directed toward prevention interventions; and similarly, evaluation of public health and clinical interventions is not possible. "If our outcome is to reduce death by suicide for this population, that question is automatically off the table [for this population] because we do not include sexual orientation and gender identity in administrative datasets like we do for other populations." He noted that this affects even community-based interventions and urged making administrative datasets inclusive. The discussion at the end of this panel briefly returned to the absence of mortality data for sexual and gender minority veterans; there, Blosnich said, to rectify this, "we are currently trying to train death investigators to gather information about sexual orientation and gender identity;" he also said that while the National Violent Death Reporting System at the CDC does have fields for sexual orientation and gender identity, these fields are left blank about 80 percent of the time.

BLACK AMERICAN MEN AND PROVIDER ROLE STRAIN

Suicide among young Black men in America has increased in recent years, said Joe. He pointed to provider role strain—the societal alignment of economic success and masculinity—as one social determinant of health that may be a significant driver of this increase.

Joe presented on social determinants of health as they affect rates of suicide among young Black American men; he focused particularly on the effects of normative cultural expectations of men to play the role of provider. He began by reviewing data showing a marked increase in suicide morbidity among in young Black men in the United States. He then defined provider role strain and discussed its significance as a social determinant of suicide risk for younger Black American men in particular. He closed the paper with a discussion of how this data might be used to reduce risk of suicide in the Black veteran population.

Joe reiterated that different ethnic groups can face different and higher risks for suicide. Such differences, he noted, suggest the need for different strategies for intervention and prevention. As an example, he highlighted differences between Black Americans and White Americans in the general population, noting that for White Americans, the risk of suicide increases with age while for Black Americans, risk of suicide peaks by age 35 and then declines with age.

Zeroing in on the suicide rates for Black Americans, Joe pointed to data that show that young Black men are disproportionately at risk, with firearms as the primary method used for all ages. These data include rates of suicide by sex, which are significantly higher for men than women between the ages of 10 and 84 within the Black population (Centers for Disease Control, Web-based Injury Statistics Query and Reporting System, 2021, 2022). It also includes rates of suicide by age; suicide is one of the top 10 causes of death for Black Americans (of both sexes) from ages 5–34. Within that young age group, firearms are the primary method (Centers for Disease Control, Web-based Injury Statistics Query and Reporting System, 2021).

This pattern, Joe noted, has "great social consequences" and should be considered when thinking about how to prevent suicide. He observed that this loss of the "very young" has different consequences than suicide among White Americans, which trends older and results in the loss of past generations. "Among Black Americans, we are losing future generations"— "future contributors to society." Joe cites one response to this phenomenon, *Ring the Alarm: The Crisis of Black Youth Suicide in America* (2019), a report from the Congressional Black Caucus Emergency Taskforce on Black Youth Suicide and Mental Health made in an effort to draw attention to this situation. This report draws on data from trend analysis and shows that for most age groups, from 2001–2015, the rate of suicide for White Americans was higher than for Black Americans, with one exception, Joe explained; in the 12 and under age group, the rate of suicide for Black children was higher than that for White children (Bridge et al., 2018). The suicide rate for Black children increased 86 percent, and for Hispanic children by 3 percent, while the rate for their White counterparts decreased 32 percent (Bridge et al., 2015). Joe noted that recent data show the continuation of this increase in rates of suicide among Black children, up 123 percent from 2010 to 2022 (Centers for Disease Control, Web-based Injury Statistics Query and Reporting System, 2022).

Joe then turned to factors that might be contributing to this: "What is it about being Black and male that increases their risk for suicide?" He pointed to the concept of "role strain," defined as "the objective difficulty, and cognitive appraisals of such difficulty, that people in highly valued life roles . . . experience" (Bowman, 2006, p. 120) in meeting "the social and cultural standards" set out for a particular social role. Provider role strain is one variation of this, Joe continues. "For Black men, the inability to fulfill the roles of the patriarch and economic provider . . . has an impact on their perception of their inability to meet the social and cultural standards of what it means to be a man." Joe noted that within the Black community, these include the ability to provide, procreate, and protect. While such normative ideas of masculinity are tied to basic notions of the American Dream, attempts by Black males to adhere to these roles are complicated by racial discrimination, he observed. He stated that Black men tend to blame themselves as individuals, rather than systemic bias and racial discrimination, for any failure to fulfill roles that are often defined by cultural expectations.

There is very little research on masculinity and how the inability to fulfill expected roles might impact suicidal behaviors, Joe points out, but provider role strain might be considered a social determinant whose indicators also point to increased risk of suicide. Drawing on data from the National Survey of American Life (NSAL), a national household probability sample of 5,181 Black respondents aged 18 years and older, conducted between February 2001 and June 2003 (Jackson et al., 2004), Joe identified some variables to measure provider role strain that might, in turn, function as predictors for an increased risk for suicide ideation and suicide attempts among Black men. These variables include food insufficiency (i.e., regularly not having enough to eat), material hardship (i.e., not meeting basic needs, including housing and utilities), and work status (including not just unemployment, but employed and not earning enough), Joe clarified. He explained, food insufficiency indicated that the individual was twice as likely to think about suicide; similarly, those not in the labor force were twice as prone to suicidal ideation. Odds ratio analysis showed that the lower the level of material hardship, the lower the level of risk for suicide, but not significantly so. Similarly, when predicting suicide attempts, material hardship and food insufficiency did not show statistical significance. However, Joe pointed out, in the area of work status, being unemployed or not in the labor force did elevate risk for suicide attempts within this sample of Black American males by at least four times. These data show how "social determinants are playing a role in the Black male's risk for suicide."

Using the data in the NSAL sample, Joe also made what he called the American Dream Index, a subset of the group who was beginning to achieve homeownership and other achievements tied to normative sociocultural expectations of the male role as provider, patriarch, and protector. He reported that analysis here showed that the lower the mean score, the less likely the individual is to achieve the American Dream and more likely to either consider or attempt suicide.

Joe noted that, as a whole, these data reveal social determinants of health for Black Americans that must be considered when working with veteran populations. One example he points to is the high rate of firearms use in suicide among both Black and veteran populations.

Joe also emphasizes veterans' vulnerability to factors associated with provider role strain in the period of transition from active duty to non-active duty and out of the armed services. This shift away from a sense of "great belonging" and relatively straightforward access to assistance has the potential, he noted, to leave veterans feeling "disconnected, uncertain, and without purpose." These feelings are also associated with provider role strain, Joe noted, as veterans figure out a new role and job. He speaks of "the importance of matching career and opportunity once [veterans] leave that very skilled setting of armed services." More generally, Joe said, "this combination of factors" that contribute to provider role strain and also are present in the moment of veterans' transition out of active duty "must be considered for any community-level suicide prevention strategy particularly for Black Americans."

DISCUSSION

The discussion, moderated by Ramchand, covered questions of data, the impact of military culture on expectations for Black males, discrimination as a social determinant, and why Black American children seem to be at increasingly higher risk for suicide.

Joe addressed the possibility that hyper masculine military culture might intensify self-perceived expectations about what the role of a man should for Black men more than White men; he commented, "I would expect to see a hardening of the adherence to . . . normative expectations among those entering the military." Joe continued that he would not suggest that there are differences between ethnic groups (including Black and White men) in terms of how this role intensifies in the military; but, he said, younger generations of Black Americans are adhering to broader American cultural norms, and "now we are beginning to see a rise [of suicide] particularly among younger Blacks." So, he reiterated, entering into the military would harden normative expectations and pressure to meet them.

Discussion of these two presentations also engaged with the theme of discrimination as a social determinant. Acknowledging that addressing discrimination from a policy position is a "long game," Ramchand observed that in the short term at the individual and community levels, "we can address the *stressors* that discrimination causes. But how can we, in the short term, address from the social determinants' perspective, some of these discriminatory practices?" Blosnich mentioned very recent discriminatory legislation passed in Florida, the so-called "Don't Say Gay" bill, and pointed to the importance of mobilizing communities and helping people to find movements that work against this sort of legislation. Blosnich commented that in addition to fighting for change in and of itself, being a part of such communities can also be a way of "processing how society currently is, and feeling you can do something." Joe observed that "we know [discrimination] is a social determinant" and so it is important to understand how it impact an individual's experience. He added that policies and practices that "make people feel of less value" will "exacerbate the stress response" and increase risk of factors that lead to suicide or serving as a "precipitating trigger" that confirms a self-perception of not mattering. Joe specified that addressing this at the individual level means helping others navigate discrimination, while efforts at the community level should "try to eliminate that experience."

The final topic of the question-and-answer session was possible reasons behind the increase in suicide risk among Black youth. Joe explored one reason within the "multifactorial explanation:" changing cultural expectations. He noted that Black children are subject to cultural expectations that are not so different than White children, "so why would they not be at risk" in the same way (i.e., at higher risk)? These cultural expectations may put younger generations of Black Americans at risk in ways that are different than earlier generations, who were not subject to the same cultural expectations. "There has been a change in cultural expectations between the generations," and so now we are seeing a corresponding increase in rates of suicide morbidity, Joe suggested. He added that some protective factors have waned "or are no longer as protective." As Black individuals become subject to cultural expectations around individual achievement and the American Dream—"I should be able to achieve as much as everyone else"—Joe said, they may encounter obstacles that are not the result of individual factors but social determinants, but not see these obstacles as such. As a result, individuals internalize a sense of personal responsibility for outcomes that are actually largely structurally determined. This mismatch can put individuals at higher risk for suicide morbidity; "I think that is what is happening with Black children nowadays," Joe concludes.

5

Community Interventions for Suicide Prevention and Support for Veterans

The second session of the symposium featured panelists discussing various community interventions to address social, cultural, and economic determinants of suicide risk, said Strauman. The first panel focused on coalitions and interventions focused specifically on suicide prevention; the second panel featured presentations on specific points of intervention—housing, and place more generally—and on a collaborative method of intervention, all through the lens of addressing social determinants of health in order to lower the risk of suicide among veterans. The second panel of this session occurred on the second day of the symposium and is described in the next chapter.

Speakers in the first panel included Nicola Winkel (Arizona Coalition for Military Families), who reported on prevention efforts in Arizona. Joseph Simonetti (VA Rocky Mountain Mental Illness Research, Education, and Clinical Center [MIRECC] for Suicide Prevention) discussed community-driven firearm suicide prevention. And the panel's third speaker, Debra Houry (Centers for Disease Control and Prevention), described the CDC's technical package on suicide prevention.

UPSTREAM PREVENTION BY ADDRESSING SOCIAL DETERMINANTS OF HEALTH

> Winkel discussed "Be Connected," one state-level organization that focuses on upstream prevention of suicide by supporting community-based efforts to address adverse social determinants of health. She spoke of the importance of a "coordinated ecosystem of support" that involved partnerships across systems and sectors to address adverse social determinants of health at multiple levels.

The Arizona Coalition for Military Families and the Governor's Challenge

Winkel spoke about veteran suicide prevention through state-level support of community prevention efforts. She discussed the work of the Arizona Coalition for Military Families (ACMF), a state-level "public-private partnership and collective impact initiative," established in 2009, whose current program Be Connected, established in 2017, serves Arizona service members, veterans, and their families. Be Connected focuses on upstream prevention of suicide across all social determinants of health. She also briefly discussed the Governor's Challenge, a national program similarly aimed at coordinating community efforts in suicide prevention.

Winkel noted that the ACMF focuses on "all helpers, organizations, and communities to create a coordinated ecosystem of support." The program Be Connected has provided resources and care navigation to service members, veterans, family members, and helpers in more than 70,000 encounters over the past five years. Winkel described the program as a "team of teams," including partnerships across systems and sectors, and involving a host of participants: people who answer the support line phones, care navigators, career navigators, community outreach navigators, people fostering community engagement, and the risk reduction operations team.

Be Connected grew out of an earlier program run by the ACMF, Be Resilient. That program, in place from 2011 to 2013, focused on members of the Arizona National Guard, which had the highest rates of suicide in the history of the organization for three years running (2008–2010), Winkel explained. In the three years Be Resilient was in place, there were no suicides within the Arizona National Guard. Building on this experience and knowledge gained, the ACMF developed Be Connected, an expanded program meant to serve the whole military population, she said. Since 2020, the ACMF, with technical assistance from the CDC, has been working to develop a data tool that enables "a proactive focus on engaging those at highest risk," she said.

Winkel explained how several features of the Be Connected program were part of this effort to proactively engage those at highest risk. The program is comprehensive in its scope, engaging with "all aspects of the military veteran and family experience" including social determinants of health, and points throughout the life course of the individual, she said. It is similarly inclusive in terms of people served and helpers involved, Winkel noted. This breadth extends to its collaborations with partners representing a range of public and private sectors, she said. Such breadth leads to "greater impact." Winkel pointed to agencies and organizations in states and communities the country, including the Governor's Challenge and Mayor's Challenges, that are engaging in similar efforts and, significantly, "engaging with their counterparts in other states, territories, [and] communities" to strengthen local efforts. Winkel noted that the ACMF has worked with the Service Members, Veterans, and their Families Technical Assistance Center for more than a decade, providing technical assistance to every other state and territory nationally during that time.

Winkel also described Be Connected as rooted in a public health approach that integrates "crisis response, treatment, and proactive prevention." She commented that this also means "not using the exact same approach for every service member, veteran, and family member" but instead adopting "an upstream prevention model" that has a "layered approach of universal, selective, and indicated efforts" and seeks to provide support before a situation becomes urgent. The goal of Be Connected is to "provide earlier intervention to reach people all across the stress continuum," which gives "more opportunity to connect with people and practice prevention strategies," Winkel said.

Winkel pointed to a current project guiding the work of the ACMF and Be Connected—as a grantee of the CDC around developing a logic model that allows for "outcome evaluation of our upstream prevention approaches and our risk reduction strategies." The logic model allows for evaluation of short-term and intermediate-term goals that contribute to the "ultimate goal" of reducing death by suicide by improving social determinants of health, she said.

Winkel reviewed some universal strategies employed by Be Connected to improve social determinants of health. These include:

- Inclusive messaging. Winkel noted that the messaging around Be Connected is inclusive in two vectors, who it serves and at what point a person might draw on those services. Messaging emphasizes that "we are here to serve everyone who was touched by . . . military service and those who are helping them." Additionally, materials focus not just on "active crisis" but connecting earlier on the stress continuum.

- A public service campaign. Be Connected partnered with the Arizona Broadcasting Association to put out TV and radio ads, and public service announcements statewide.
- A support line that provides resource and care navigation. Winkel reports that the support line team has had more than 70,000 encounters in the last five years. An evaluation of callers revealed that about 85 percent were at "low acuity" category of risk; 14.5 percent needed more intensive and ongoing support; about 0.5 percent were in the crisis category, meaning that the program was effectively reaching people pre-crisis.

Selective strategies of prevention target higher-risk segments of the population, said Winkel. "If you know who the segments are, how do you then translate that into a functional program or approach?" Winkel noted that Be Connected has taken a proactive approach that involves identifying high-risk groups, developing and implementing targeted programs, collecting data and evaluating outcomes, and iterating in ways that are responsive to that data and "lessons learned." One example of this that Winkel pointed to a project run with the State Department of Veterans' Services where that agency proactively refers veterans with a known or potential disability directly to the Be Connected team, which then connects them to resources needed for issues outside their disability claim. Another example Winkel gave was developing projects that support service members as they transition out of the military; these include programs focused on support navigation, mentorship, and food insecurity.

Indicated strategies employed by Be Connected work at the individual level, Winkel said. This includes training and equipping "helpers" in the community "because they are the ones who are best positioned to identify and connect and support" veterans. Be Connected has trained more than 6,000 people in resource navigation in Arizona, she reported. It is part of "an ongoing effort to ensure that we have . . . thousands of open doors across the state of people who are willing, ready, and able to help get someone connected."

COMMUNITY-DRIVEN EFFORTS TO PREVENT FIREARM SUICIDE

Recent data show a promising increase in community-based efforts to prevent suicide by firearm, Simonetti reported. Such community efforts are important and impactful because they have the potential to reach veterans outside of a clinical setting, and to normalize conversations about firearm safety and mental health within that community.

Simonetti presented on community-based efforts to prevent suicide by firearm, first discussing why these efforts are critical in solving the larger problem of firearm suicide. "There is a longstanding acknowledgement of the fundamental role that communities play [in] determining health outcomes generally," noted Simonetti. With respect to firearm injuries in particular, community interventions may reach where health care systems cannot, constrained as they are by "important limitations," present in a system's reach, credibility, resources, and focus. First, health care systems are limited by the simple fact that they "can only intervene on the people they see," said Simonetti. He noted that in the VA, the clinical population is less than half of the total U.S. veteran population. Second, health care systems "have unique credibility" within this population, Simonetti said, which is not necessarily better or worse than the credibility afforded to other potential messengers, but truly different. As such, "community efforts have a unique opportunity to talk about firearm suicide prevention in a way that clinical systems do not." Third, hospital systems and clinics have time constraints, competing priorities, and "varying levels of comfort and . . . knowledge" among the clinical staff. Fourth, community-based outreach allows for a focus on "some of the fundamental factors driving suicide outcomes" as theorized by the "socio-ecological model" rather than those identified in the bio-medical approach.

Simonetti noted the promising increase of prevention work at the community level over the past 10 years, and turned to a short overview of some of these efforts. The first was work through the VA by Mohatt to build "community-driven and community-based infrastructure for suicide prevention in rural areas." One aspect of this project is to develop coalitions of veterans who work to "normalize and reinforce conversations about firearms as well as suicide risk at the community level," especially in rural areas that are disproportionately at risk for suicide by firearm, said Simonetti. As one example, he referenced a veteran coalition in Montana that hosted a suicide prevention table at a local firearm show.

Providing firearm storage options for at-risk veterans is another area where community-based programs might have more success than clinical practice settings, said Simonetti. Temporarily storing firearms outside of the home can protect at-risk veterans and others, he noted, and reported that clinical practice data as well as "preliminary data from national studies" show that "veterans do in fact hold on to firearms for other individuals at risk or store their own firearms out of their homes when they are going through really hard times." Simonetti pointed to the Armory Project, a Louisiana-based coalition of firearm retailers and VA researchers who offer firearm storage options to at-risk veterans.

While the VA and other health care systems might have limitations, Simonetti said, there are still ways of contributing "to this conversation on firearm injury prevention and suicide risk at the community level." The VA has partnered with the American Foundation for Suicide Prevention and the National Shooting Sports Foundation to co-develop materials on firearm injury prevention that are disseminated through "a variety of firearm industry and community suicide prevention channels."

Simonetti also pointed to "a number of organic initiatives" independent of the VA and other health care systems that do similar work. One such program is Walk the Talk America, a program run by "really dedicated individuals" in the firearm community whose stated goal is to raise awareness about guns, mental health, and suicide prevention. Those who run the program "know this role better than most people." Another program is the Overwatch Project, which encourages participants (including service members as well as veterans) to ask "hard and . . . uncomfortable questions about suicide risk in an effort to support their peers and normalize these conversations about . . . the link between firearm access and suicide risk." All of these programs are dedicated to raising awareness and normalizing conversation around suicide.

One of the central challenges to the prevention of suicide by firearm is striking a balance between the protection of oneself in a crisis by limiting access to firearms and, on the other hand, "a common perception in the United States that one needs to maintain ready access to a firearm for protection from other people," Simonetti said. Approximately two-thirds of veterans who own firearms keep their firearms in case they need protection from other people. Simonetti pointed to public service announcements as one intervention strategy that can reduce the stigma around "making changes to one's firearm access" as a way of protecting oneself or others; he commented that while such messaging may not be obviously community based, it plays a key role in normalizing conversation about the link firearms and suicide risk at both national and community level. He noted that such prevention efforts have been focused on increasing awareness about this link; one opportunity for development is community-driven efforts that focus on "the other side of the equation," that is, "helping at-risk persons navigate their concerns about victimization risk and whether or not they truly need to maintain firearm access in these situations," said Simonetti.

Simonetti summed up his presentation by reiterating the affordances of community-driven intervention efforts: to extend beyond clinical settings; to leverage the expertise of those within these communities; to identify and harness resources within the community that might only be known about by its members; and to normalize discussion about the link between firearms and suicide risk within the community. This normalization of conversation about this topic "can ideally change the risk parameters of the communities themselves," Simonetti concluded.

THE CDC TECHNICAL PACKAGE ON SUICIDE PREVENTION

> The CDC's technical package on suicide prevention includes evidence-based strategies meant to help communities and states focus on priorities with the greatest potential for favorable outcomes, Houry said. These strategies include (1) strengthen economic supports; (2) strengthen access to and delivery of suicide care; (3) create protective environments; (4) promote connectedness; (5) teach coping and problem-solving skills; (6) identify and support people at risk for suicide; and (7) lessen harms and prevent future risk.

Houry gave an overview of the CDC's technical package on suicide prevention, "Preventing Suicide: A Technical Package of Policy, Programs, and Practices" (https://sprc.org/news/preventing-suicide-technical-package-policy-programs-practices, 2017). She began by sketching the criteria for inclusion in a technical package. Following this, she detailed the seven strategies at the core of the CDC technical package on suicide prevention.

This technical package includes "strategies based on the best available evidence to help communities and states focus on priorities with the greatest potential to prevent a public health problem"—in this case, the risk of suicide, Houry explained. Each program, practice, or policy included in the technical package has to meet at least one of the listed criteria, she continued:

- Be a meta-analysis or systematic review.
- Show impact on suicide or significant impact on risk or protective factors for suicide.
- Show that there was evidence from at least one rigorous evaluation showing preventative effects on suicide or significant impact on risk or protective factors for suicide.

Houry emphasized that this range is in response to the fact that suicide itself is not caused by a single factor, "and therefore will not be prevented by any single intervention." The technical package gathers "prevention strategies and approaches that address the range of suicide risk and protective factors at the individual, relationship, community, and societal levels." She said, "preventing suicide requires strategies at all levels of society." Houry also noted, "by building on community strengths and focusing not just on treatment but on this coordinated approach to prevention, we can meet the immediate needs of those already affected today while preventing future risks."

The seven strategies of suicide prevention central to this technical package include strengthen economic supports (1); strengthen access to and delivery of suicide care (2); create protective environments (3); promote connectedness (4); teach coping and problem-solving skills (5); identify and support people at risk for suicide (6); and lessen harms and prevent future risk (7).

The first strategy, strengthen economic supports, responds to the link between financial wellbeing and risk of suicide, Houry noted. She explained, "Strengthening household financial security provides individuals with financial means to lessen stress and hardships associated with . . . unanticipated financial problems."

Strengthening access to and delivery of suicide care can take a number of forms, Houry said. These might include implementing laws that require insurers to cover mental health conditions on par with physical health conditions; "reducing provider shortages in underserved areas through financial incentive programs and expanding the reach of telehealth;" and developing health care systems that emphasize patient-centered care (including continuity of care, continuous quality improvement, and promotion of equity for all patients).

Creating protective environments by making positive changes can have a major impact on individuals, Houry said. Such changes might include reducing access to lethal means, including focused intervention at suicide hotspots; implementing policies aimed at reducing excessive alcohol use; and implementing organizational policies and values such as the promotion of seeking health care, changing social norms, and bringing awareness to helping services. As an example of the latter, Houry pointed to the U.S. Air Force's community-based Suicide Prevention Program, a required training associated with a decline in suicide of more than 30 percent as well as declines in family violence and homicides.

A sense of connectedness can decrease isolation and increase a sense of belonging, both protective factors against suicide, Houry said. She pointed to peer norm programs, which "can normalize protective factors such as health-seeking and reaching out to trusted adults." Sources of Strength is a school-based program; it is associated with "improvements in adaptive norms, connectedness to adults, and school engagement." This program has been adapted in the Air Force, where it is called Wingmen Connect. Urban greening initiatives and group exercise are other examples, Houry said.

Teaching necessary coping and problem-solving skills is the fifth strategy Houry discussed. One domain is social-emotional learning, she said; programs in this domain can help children and youth to "develop and strengthen communication and problem-solving skills, resolve problems and relationships at school and with peers," and can help them address "other negative influences such as substance abuse, which can be associated with suicide," said Houry. She pointed to the Youth Aware of Mental Health Program as one example of this kind of education, with a focus on teaching children and youth about positive mental health practices. Another domain is parenting skills; Houry noted that The Incredible Years is an example of a training program for parents, teachers, and children[1] that has been shown to "decrease risk factors from suicide such as substance abuse and to increase protective factors, including emotion regulation and social competence."

One aspect of the strategy of identifying and supporting people at risk for suicide is "gatekeeper training," where teachers, coaches, primary care providers, and other community members learn to identify and effectively respond to people who may be at risk of suicide, said Houry. Her example here is the Applied Suicide Intervention Skills Training, which "helps counselors, emergency workers, and others to identify and connect with individuals at risk for suicide and assist with linking individuals to resources." Evaluations have shown a reduction in suicide attempts in counties implementing gatekeeper training. She noted that crisis intervention is another effective part of this strategy, with services like Lifeline making "space or time" between suicidal ideation and harmful behaviors. Another component of this strategy, Houry said, is psychotherapy focused on building problem solving and emotional regulation skills, including the program Improving Mood-Promoting Access to Collaborative Treatment. This strategy also includes treatment focused on preventing reattempts, which is an "especially important" element, she noted. Such intervention might take a number of different forms of follow-up contacts over varying periods of time.

The seventh strategy Houry described was lessening harms and preventing future risk, meant to prevent suicide contagion; this involves "postvention approaches . . . implemented after a suicide has taken place" to support those who know someone who died by suicide. The StandBy Response Service is an initiative by the Australian government that provides support to individuals and communities impacted by suicide, Houry noted. She also pointed to "safe reporting and messaging" about suicide that can prevent suicide risk through the inclusion of stories of hope and resilience, prevention messages, and links to helping resources.

Houry concluded by noting that the CDC is providing funding to groups in 11 states to support the implementation of "this comprehen-

---

[1] Other important work to highlight includes the Creating Opportunities for Personal Empowerment (COPE) cognitive-behavioral therapy-based program for children, teens and young adults, which has more than 20 studies to support its efficacy in reducing depression, suicidal ideation, alcohol use and anxiety, and improving healthy behaviors. It is being implemented in primary care practices with reimbursement as well as primary and secondary schools and universities.

sive approach" outlined in the technical package, with several participant organizations focusing on veteran suicide prevention. She also pointed to the Veteran Suicide Prevention Evaluation programs, which helps to build "evaluation capacity for upstream suicide prevention programs."

DISCUSSION

Simonetti began the discussion by addressing the challenge of finding effective, "shared" language to use around firearm safety within the firearm community and veteran population. He pointed to data showing that a difference in how clinicians and firearm owners define or think about "what firearm safety really is." He noted that there are some trainings around "cultural competence in firearm injury prevention;" he also urged talking with members of the community—"whether that is veteran engagement at a local facility [or] walking into a firearm retail store and having a conversation with somebody"—as a way of developing a shared language.

Winkel spoke to the importance of "an ecosystem approach" to prevention intervention that provides mental health support for families of veterans as well as veterans themselves. Inclusive messaging is key to communicating the possibility of this, she noted.

Answering a question about the intersection of change to COVID-19 and veteran suicide, Houry said that thus far, there is no evidence of an increase in suicide deaths during the pandemic. However, she said, there has been an increase in risk factors, including economic instability, unemployment, social isolation, disruption of access to treatment. She advocated for prevention of suicide deaths as a result of these increased risk factors; such prevention could include "continuing to focus resiliency, connectedness, preventing ACEs [adverse childhood experiences]" and also attending particularly to those groups where mental health distress has been shown to increase (including underrepresented minority groups and essential workers, including health care providers and health care workers), Houry said.

Simonetti noted the promise of on-site storage options being developed within the firearm retail community, but observed that there is no codified approach or set of resources for engaging with shops to promote this. He pointed to the VA in New Orleans, and across Louisiana, as an instance of an agency engaging with gun shops on this topic. From those conversations, he said, they have seen the importance of having someone from the firearm community. He mentioned that some of the main challenges are how the operator of the on-site storage facility would know when to give the gun back, and what their liability would be around that transfer. Later in the discussion, Simonetti also spoke to the complexity of messaging in striking a balance between protecting oneself from suicide risk and from violence from others; misinformation can skew the message, he said, but Simonetti noted that he worries more about the way two different people might receive and internalize the same message in different ways. He pointed to the importance of developing a shared language, communicating risk in a way that all will hear and understand.

Brenner, the panel moderator, posed the question of how best to implement the strategies and approaches discussed in the technical package and tool kits from various programs discussed by Houry and Winkel. Winkel commented on the essential nature of community groups partnering with programs and agencies that can provide technical assistance, helping to "translate information and intent into a plan" and building in evaluation of outcomes, as well. Houry pointed to the CDC resource Violence Prevention in Practice, which goes through some of the steps involved with implementing aspects of the technical package. Both spoke to the importance of helping community groups evaluate, choose, implement, and sustain specific intervention strategies based on the needs of the community they are serving.

Brenner also raised the question of challenges communities can face in partnering with state governments (whether programs or agencies) if there is not an alignment between the organization and the government or where community and state or federal leaders are not moving in the same direction. Winkel emphasized the hard work involved in building partnerships, especially across sectors and communities

6

Community Interventions for Varied Applications in Housing, Health, and Safety

The final panel of the first day, and the second panel of the second session, featured three presenters speaking about various forms and applications of community interventions. Jack Tsai (VA Homeless Programs Office and University of Texas) spoke about how housing and homelessness are related to suicide and the impact VA programs to alleviate homelessness have had on suicide risk. Holly Raffle (Ohio University) discussed the importance of collaboration, focusing on a range of ways that community-based coalitions might effectively address prevention of veteran suicide. Charles Branas (Columbia University) presented on the impact place can have on health, including the importance of place-based interventions in preventing suicide.

HOUSING AND HOMELESSNESS

While data show a link between suicide and homelessness, this link is likely via shared upstream risk factors, Tsai remarked. Perhaps because of this, he said, there is evidence that some VA homeless programs are having an impact on suicide risk, including the program Supportive Services for Veteran Families (SSVF).

Homeless populations—both veterans and other adults—have a high risk for suicide, Tsai noted, citing in particular a systematic review by Adam Hoffberg et al. (2018) that shows higher rates of both suicide attempts and suicide deaths among homeless veterans than veterans who are not homeless. Tsai also pointed to a study he led that found a "stronger association between homelessness and suicide among veterans" than non-veterans; while it is not clear why this is, he said, he noted that there are "upstream factors that are . . . common to both" and that these shared factors may be the reason for this stronger association in veterans (Tsai & Cao, 2019). These factors include being male; low socioeconomic status; mental illness; lack of social support; substance use disorders; chronic medical conditions; and adverse childhood events. Past experience of homelessness is also a predictor of homelessness, just as a family history of suicide and suicidal attempts are predictors of suicide, he said. One study looking at the timing around suicide risk and homelessness suggests that suicidal behavior often precedes homelessness (Culhane et al., 2019), Tsai reported. "This is important in terms of intervention and planning of services," he noted.

Tsai then turned to an overview of VA homeless programs, particularly the Supportive Services for Veteran Families (SSVF) program, and their impact on suicide risk and mortality. The VA offers a range of homeless programs that serve more than 100,000 veterans a year. He referenced a study that compares homeless veterans who participated in a VA homeless program to homeless veterans who did not, and shows that "use of any VA homeless program was associated with 6 percent reduction in all-cause mortality and 21 percent reduction in suicide mortality" (Montgomery et al., 2021). The study also shows that use of additional homeless programs yields "an incremental benefit," Tsai reported, with each additional program used reducing risk for all-cause mortality by a further 7 percent and suicide mortality by 19 percent. This study "really shows that homeless services do address social determinants of physical and mental health, and that [these services] reduce death overall" and especially suicide death, he summarized.

The SSVF program in the VA funds community grantees to provide services to homeless veterans. Tsai noted that this has the advantage of connecting veterans with providers who can, in turn, connect them to resources from the community as well as the VA. The program has two components: the Rapid Re-Housing Program, and the homeless prevention component, including temporary financial assistance (TFA). Both focus on "providing brief case management" and offer short-term assistant with rent and utilities; the former focuses on veterans who are homeless, with the goal of re-housing, while the latter focuses on veterans who are in imminent risk of homelessness. Program data on the return rate to homelessness show that, overall, one year out, more than 85 percent of veterans who use the SSVF have not returned to homeless programs, Tsai reported.

The TFA component of the SSVF has been shown to reduce health care service use and health care costs, mostly for inpatient costs, where there was a $372 reduction per quarter, Tsai said. He noted that the reduction in inpatient costs means that veterans reduced need for "intensive services" for mental health and medical needs, which provides evidence for temporary financial assistance as an effective intervention. Tsai pointed to a separate study that found that "temporary financial assistance increases housing stability as well." However, a randomized controlled trial is needed to conclude effectiveness, he said.

"Studies have shown that participation in VA homeless program is associated with reduced risk of death, including suicide death," said Tsai (Nelson et al., 2021). The SSVF program in particular is "exemplary in terms of a VA-community partnership model that can help address social determinants of health and health care costs," which can in turn impact suicide risk, he concluded.

USING A COLLABORATIVE APPROACH IN SUICIDE PREVENTION

Because suicide is a complex problem that cannot be solved in a simple way, multiple solution sets must be developed, Raffle said. Collaborative efforts can be especially effective in this. Collaboration is most successful when participants consider whether they have the capacity for it; when there are inter-institutional supports; and when it is approached as a skill that can be learned.

Suicide is a "wicked problem"—meaning a complex problem with more than one solution that are often "not solvable" in a simple way, Raffle said. "We solve and re-solve [wicked problems] again and again." As such, the problem demands "multiple solution sets." Raffle noted the effectiveness of a collaborative approach in suicide prevention work in producing multiple solution sets. She pointed to the Substance Abuse and Mental Health Services Administration's 2016 declaration that "collaboration among prevention professionals across behavioral health fields has the potential to reduce suicide rates."

There are many different ways of working together, Raffle noted. She illustrated this by way of a continuum showing stages of collaborative relationships, where participants are least to most enmeshed. These stages range from "immuring" (i.e., working primarily on one's own) and "networking" to "collaboration" and "integration" (i.e., fully merging operations, structures, budgets) (Mashek, 2015). Organizations and individuals must "pick the best way to collaborate that works for your given situation," she said. To this end, Raffle recommended a decision process based around three key questions: Can I do it? Will it work? Is it worth it? to support groups in deciding which type of collaborative relationship was appropriate or the best-fit scenario given the local circumstances. She compared this process, based on work by E. Scott Gellar, to the decision-making process involving the evaluation, selection, and implementation of specific interventions. Asking these questions can help participants in multiple situations: the critical work of evaluating strategies and selecting those that fit the capacity of those involved and that are "culturally responsive and sustainable" within the community as well as determining the level of collaboration that is required for any individual project, she said.

Raffle emphasized that collaborations evolve as the work continues (though she noted that it is not necessarily a goal for partnerships to move from less integrated to more integrated). Collaboration is a learned skill, she stressed, and as such, requires supports that facilitate this learning. Key areas where this takes place are capacity, inter-institutional supports, and a practice mindset, Raffle said. The latter describes approaching collaboration as "something that you constantly have to practice in order to get better," she said. Raffle explained that as organizations work together, they can more fully develop an understanding of what collaboration involves and how to do it more successfully.

The first of these three key areas, *capacity*, describes developing organizational ability to connect, share, or coordinate efforts in a collaborative relationship, Raffle said. The question "Can I do it" becomes, "Do we have the capacity to work together at this time?" Organizational capacity can change over time, whether due to external factors or growth through accumulated internal experience, she noted. Illustrating the former, Raffle pointed to the example of two organizations who were at the cooperation stage on the collaboration continuum when the COVID-19 pandemic disrupted normal operations and forced them to pull back from cooperation to the "immuring" stage as they devoted time and resources to basic functioning within their own organization. She noted that once the two organizations figured out those changes to some degree, they had the capacity to resume their cooperative work. As to the latter, Raffle noted that collaborations might start with small—with a networking meeting, for example, or the establishment of a clear communication channel—and evolve slowly, as specific capacities are developed.

Raffle's model connects *inter-institutional supports*, the second key area, with the evaluative question "Will it work?" Collaboration will work only if there is "support from our authorizing environment." The more integrated the partnership, the more institutional support is needed, explained Raffle. Sometimes, she said, collaborations fail not because people do not have the capacity or lack the desire, "but because they do not have the support structures or do not honor [the idea that] support structures are necessary."

The third key area, approaching collaboration through *a growth mindset*, links with the evaluative question "Is it worth it?" in Raffle's model. She emphasized the emotional aspect of collaboration; referencing a model by Pat Collarbone that charts a typical up-and-down emotional trajectory that moves from initial interest through frustration and despair, to optimism and hope, to commitment (2009). Raffle notes that often when people begin collaborating, they make collective impact their goal when they might be more successful starting with a less intensive collaborative relationship (e.g., networking), with the aim of building from there. Collective impact is an important strategy in our toolkits, she noted, but, "It takes time to get to the degree of collaboration on the continuum that is necessary for collective impact."

Raffle then outlined four tips for practitioners looking to collaborate. The first is to observe what organizations, programs, and coalitions already exist in the community, and look for ways of joining. "Do not start something new if you do not have to." The second is to have a sense of collaborating partners' agendas and capacities, which are likely different than one's own. "Know your space but be willing to listen and learn from others." This includes, for example, being aware of the different knowledge, skills, and attitudes that might be required for population prevention versus those required for treatment and recovery, Raffle said.

The third tip Raffle offered is to recognize that collaboration is a learned skill whose practitioners require supports. "Embed training opportunities about how to collaborate and how to lead collaborations into your funding opportunities," she recommends. The fourth tip is to keep in mind that "collaboration is an intentional practice" that takes time—often years—to see collaborative efforts come to fruition, she says, and financial investments should be planned accordingly.

PLACE-BASED INTERVENTIONS

Place—the everyday environment of one's daily life—is a social determinant of health, Branas said. Several studies have shown the connection between vacancy and abandonment in urban areas, and gun violence; interventions that "clean and green" these areas have been shown to result in decreased gun violence and other positive outcomes. These are upstream treatments that can have a wide-ranging impact, including in suicide prevention.

Branas discussed the importance of place—the "surroundings and environments that we experience every day"—in determining health, and reviewed several studies showing of impact of place-based interventions. He focused on the connection between vacancy and abandonment in urban areas, and gun violence. Branas explained that the everyday context people experience "all the time" (i.e., place) plays a role in determining poor health on par with genetics and "certainly more than the medical care you receive," and is also "a major predictor of good health" alongside other social determinants like access to medical care and education. Places can sometimes be "underlying reasons that the poor health is occurring in the first place." If environmental factors are not addressed, poor health will continue, he said.

Branas focused on the impact of vacancy and abandonment, illustrating this first by showing the effects of redlining in 1940s Chicago, which resulted—decades later—in neighborhoods with large numbers of vacant and abandoned properties that are caught up in the "spiral of structural racism, disinvestment, and abandonment." These properties are "really toxic to [the] health and safety" of people who live in those neighborhoods today, he said. This is true of many other cities, Branas said, and noted that the area of vacant and abandoned spaces in U.S. cities equals that of Switzerland.

Branas pointed to groups that are implementing "in situ place-based changes" that introduce inexpensive structural changes designed to help people stay in their home neighborhoods and to bring amenities to those areas. These amenities might include greening; fewer abandoned buildings; community gardens; and business improvement districts, he said. "They are very scalable and . . . also quite sustainable." Branas noted that while approaches differed between organizations, all began as "community-initiated ideas" and were co-designed based on input from the community, including concerns surrounding "environmental challenges that they could see on a daily basis . . . things like, you have to watch for yourself walking past vacant lots." He reported, "many community members came back to this thing: that if they could change something . . . it would be the vacant lots and the abandoned buildings." These places were often mentioned as the sources of fear and danger, whether because someone "might step out" or because the building was in a state of imminent collapse, Branas said. He noted that such places presented both challenges and opportunities.

Branas reviewed several studies he and his team have conducted. The first (2016) looked at what effects changing a place might have on the community around it. This study treated more than 10,000 vacant lots and abandoned buildings in Philadelphia, turning the vacant lots into green spaces as well as cleaning abandoned buildings and turning them into sites "do not detract" from the neighborhood as well as potentially livable places. Branas reported that there was significantly less gun violence and stress—as much as 39 percent less—around newly green spaces and newly fixed-up buildings. He stressed the cost effectiveness of this treatment, with every dollar spent yielding a return of as much as $300 through the reduction of gun violence, which is (a very costly event for a city . . . costly in many ways," including not just the immediate response but "the ripple effect of that violence" in neighborhoods.

A randomized trial (Branas et al., 2018; Moyer et al., 2019), also in Philadelphia, compared about 200 spaces that were "cleaned, greened, and maintained" with 200 spaces that were only cleaned and maintained, and with another 200 spaces that did not receive any treatment (until the end of the study, when all spaces were fully greened). Branas reported that gun violence around the cleaned and greened spaces went down by 29 percent in some areas. Two more ongoing studies, with treatments again in Philadelphia and also in New Orleans, are starting to show "similar reductions in gun violence—about 23 percent in and around these spaces," he said.

Branas pointed to good outcomes associated with these studies, or what he calls "win-win science" that results from the introduction of outside resources into communities. Treatments of the kind Branas described were shown to result in the reduction in gun violence and the reduction of nuisances (e.g., public drunkenness and noise complaints), he reported. These also yielded "co-benefits" that feed the reduction of gun violence, including the reduction of depression, fear, anxiety, and other mental health challenges; a higher willingness to go outside more; and a greater willingness to connect "not just . . . with the spaces but also to connect with each other."

These positive outcomes are the result in part of a "biologic response, with less stress, fear, and aggression" associated with these newly-renovated spaces, Branas reported. This also comes of the place functioning as a site where community members can connect with one another: the creation of a "positive, 'busy streets' environment"—a "visual cue" that communicates care about the space. And finally, changing vacant and abandoned places can remove the opportunity to store illegal firearms, he said. Branas pointed to other cities that have undertaken some combination of place-based research and programming—"in situ, inexpensive, scalable structural and sustainable place-based interventions." Across this group of cities, evidence shows between 6 percent and 66 percent less "violence, stress, fear, depression, sedentary behavior, and cardiovascular risks."

In his conclusion, Branas stressed three points. First, that programs that focus on place have upstream influence that can impact "the lives of more people and for longer periods of time than programs that simply focus on individuals." Second, that the everyday environment can play a role in the success of medical treatments for individuals. A "chaotic and unhealthy environment" can compromise the efficacy of such treatments. Third, that place-based changes might be thought of as treatments in and of themselves.

DISCUSSION

Timothy Strauman, moderator for this panel, posed two general questions to the three presenters. The first focused on the fact that, despite conventional wisdom and popular reporting that frames problems like homelessness, infrastructure deterioration, and despair as intractable, there are "some very clear indications" that progress can be made in addressing these "seemingly intractable problems." Strauman asked, "How do we get the word out that we can make this kind of significant progress and get the policy makers and the funders on board with these kinds of sustainable, economically viable programs that clearly are working?"

Branas identified the importance of simply "doing some really good science" that provides evidence for the impact of successful programs. This evidence might be used to raise awareness of success framed not just in terms of scientific outcomes but in terms that show these programs to have "a real return on the investment." Raffle added that her organization is working to help community groups craft "social determinants of health impact statements" as part of their work around suicide prevention, the reduction of gun violence, etc. These statements serve as guideposts as the groups make funding decisions, write requests for proposals and design programs, she said. Like a diversity impact statement, and ideally together with it, this social determinants of health impact statement can help organizations to "make decisions with those things at the forefront of mind," she said. Tsai added that getting the word out about success of programs addressing social determinants of health can help stakeholders with different priorities to understand that there are also common factors and mutual goals everyone is working toward.

Strauman then asked the panelists about their "most pleasant surprise in finding [that] community members, stakeholders, people who you thought would not be on board . . . actually were and [that] they were part of the solution?" Branas answered that his team was surprised with how many of the interventions, "at least in the research, turned out to be impactful." He reiterated the importance of involving "community voices early, because they will . . . contribute very much to the sustainability of these programs." With this kind of buy-in, Branas said, community members will be the ones "who will step forward to policy makers and leaders, and really elevate the program."

Raffle noted the need to highlight both prevention and promotion within a program. She pointed to Branas's discussion of how green spaces both promote health and have "a corresponding decrease," in this case, gun violence. She argues that rather than an "either/or" mindset, organizers adopt a "both/and" approach that allows for "exponential growth in your community-based process."

7

Reports from Interactive Session Groups

Activity on the second day of the symposium was built around six discussion groups, each focused on a specific population addressed in the previous day's presentations. Timothy Strauman (Duke University) provided a summary of several themes that emerged from the previous day's talks. These include the observation that "there are extensive data documenting that the social determinants of health in general are directly applicable to the specific challenge of reducing suicide risk in veterans." He commented one benefit of this is that as a result of this, "we can draw on that literature." The second theme is that in addition to approaching suicide prevention and management as an acute problem, adopting a broader perspective will make it possible to better "manage, reduce, and eliminate risk of suicide." Third, Strauman noted the central importance of "the intersection of multiple social forces and multiple identities," and the way that intersectionality might figure in suicide risk within a specific population. Fourth, he pointed to the fact that while factors contributing to suicide risk in veterans might seem intractable, panelists from day 1 of the symposium show collaborative efforts that "have already begun to make a difference." Fifth, and last, Strauman noted that interventions that reduce veterans' rates of suicide risk are also "effectively addressing other threats to their health and wellbeing."

Having set the stage in this way, Strauman turned to Molly Checksfield Dorries, who provided a brief overview of breakout group logistics. She explained the plan wherein each group would discuss how various adverse social determinants impact its focus population, and then "design, implement, and evaluate" a community intervention that might address these challenges specifically for the focus population. A common set of questions coordinated group discussion of these three points: population, adverse social determinant, and community intervention. These populations included older veterans, LGBTQ+ veterans, veterans living in rural communities, veterans with co-occurring mental health and substance use disorders, Black veterans, and women veterans.

OLDER VETERANS

The discussion group that focused on older veterans chose to address the adverse social determinants of legal problems, familial and social problems, and lack of access to care and transportation, the reporter for the group said. One of the challenges this group identified was a lack of trust in the VA, the health care system, and government policies—the sense that these did not have their "best interest as a priority," he noted. A program addressing this might involve "education and exposure to local resources and services from the VA and other service providers;" the reporter explained that this education could be undertaken not just by the VA itself, but by community, state, and federal offices and organizations. Local non-profits could be especially important in this work, "being the boots on the ground" and peer leadership that might connect with veterans who are unhappy with the services available through the VA, he said. The reporter said that barriers to this approach might include the credibility of the organization, especially if new and relatively unknown. The group envisioned a "holistic approach" to support, "just encompassing everything to get that veteran or their family member help," he said. The reporter said the group also discussed the importance of training first responders, including law enforcement, in crisis intervention and de-escalation. The group also discussed how crisis intervention teams value the insight from social workers or therapists because these experts provide special training for how to interact with a veteran in crisis in ways that lead to a "healthy conclusion."

LGBTQ+ VETERANS

The participant reporting for the LGBTQ+ group said that they chose to identify their own social determinant of health, and that they identified "enacted perceived, or anticipatory discrimination as a key undercurrent of a variety of problems that our population experiences." Group discussion centered the question of whether there is a need for new programs or are there existing programs that might work for LGBTQ+ communities but cannot be evaluated as such because there are no data or the programs do not reach that population.

The reporter listed a number of "different partner organizations that should be at the planning table in our community," including LGBTQ+ veteran organizations, VA peer support, as well as "nontraditional veteran spaces" like wellness centers, alternative therapies, community health care, and substance use treatment. The vision of partnership also included "bridging" LGBTQ+ care coordinators at the VA with the VA Center for Faith-Based and Neighborhood Partnerships. This collaboration would, ideally, make space in programs for "folks can be their whole selves.... Very often what we find is that LGBT+ veterans are not identifying as veterans."

While the group discussed a variety of different outreach materials, "we landed on implementing an evaluative rating scale for community organizations to assess their readiness or competency for working within the LGBT+ and veteran space." The aim was to connect patients with LGBT+ resources "and be physically and psychologically safe in those spaces." The reporter noted that this would result in "an LGBT+ care continuum, a map of vetted service providers."

One challenge the reporter mentioned was "the futility of it all." The massive scale of change needed can be daunting; she noted that one possible solution to this is to "bring this to life on a granular level, human to human" to create an important interpersonal connection. Evaluation posed another barrier; "how do you measure and evaluate if this is working if we do not have the data to begin with?" The group focused on tangible ways of evaluating progress—"number of gatekeeper trainings ... number of gun locks distributed"—as well as the rate of suicide among LGBTQ+ veterans. Uncovering the latter would involve attempts to partner with "the medical examiners' offices, vital statistics, and data from the state, the CDC, and the VA."

VETERANS IN RURAL COMMUNITIES

The reporter for the group focused on rural veterans said that they focused on logistics: "everything from firewood to broadband to access to trucks and transportation—all as vehicles for suicide prevention." The reporter identified some themes identified by the group; these included coalition building and service connection. Coalition-building might involve simply one person from the VA who "is a trusted source in a local community" that an individual might feel comfortable turning to even if they have doubts about the VA or mental health care. The group came up with the idea of building an academy that might teach how to build coalitions as well as teach skills like the ability to train others, grant writing, sustainability, capacity building, networking, he said. The group also noted that last in the coalition theme is the idea that "statewide coalitions ultimately can unify efforts across rural counties, making them more efficient" and highlighting "the fact that these broad sets of needs that individual communities have really all are still suicide prevention."

The second theme was service connection, meaning, "a sense of purpose." The reporter explained, "No matter where the veteran is and what is going on in their life, how do we help at the individual [or] community level . . . to get [people] engaged in ways that help their lives continue to make sense." Ramchand, moderating this portion of the symposium, mentioned We Got Your Six, a coalition for veteran community-based organizations as relevant to this group.

Challenges identified include volunteer burnout and varying levels of integration between service providers and communities, Strauman reported. He also noted that there seem to be challenges around limitations as to what a person who works for the VA would be able to do "in terms of helping somebody else write a grant or manage funds."

MENTAL HEALTH

The group focusing on mental health chose as their adverse social determinants, "familial and social problems with mental health . . .; not knowing the symptoms of PTSD or brain injury . . .; and, a lack of understanding," stated the reporter for the group. They also discussed "community response to the death by suicide of a veteran in the community and how it impacts other veterans; financial conditions and financial literacy for veterans; the feeling of isolation and loneliness, lack of access to care and to community; and . . . lack of access to transportation," he said.

One intervention the group developed was to start the process of transitioning from active duty to veteran earlier in a career, before the point of separation, the reporter said. Challenges identified by the group included too many options for veterans to choose from, he said. Varying quality of care was another concern, he noted, as was a lack of communication about services available. In the case of the latter, this encompassed communication *between* organizations as well as advertising messaging: "A lot of times, one place will not know what another place has to offer."

Components of this community intervention included what the reporter for the group called "the magic wand one": the removal of all barriers to access needed services. The development of a centralized and informed source of knowledge for all available services in a particular community is another component, he said. Another key aspect of this community intervention was various forms of education: training for law enforcement focused on veteran needs; education for family and friends "on what the special needs of a retiring military person might be;" and financial education for veterans. The group reporter stressed the importance of securing funding to support services, and especially legislative advocacy for funding. Another component was the use of support structures like veteran peer support networks to help with the transition; an audience participant noted that in using veteran peer specialists, the support could be "all-encompassing of the veteran instead of just recovery coaching" or support for other mental health issues. The group also included the idea of creating a storytelling space, where veterans can talk "about their process of retiring and then integrating into the civilian world," he said, adding that this can normalize conversation about this process, including concerns and issues that might have arisen.

Organizations that might be brought into this include "local mental health authorities, the VA, local nonprofits, workforce training organizations and services, and the faith-based community," the reporter for the group stated.

Ramchand noted that the chat conversation included mention of the Department of Labor's Transition Assistance Program and local chapters of the American Foundation for Suicide Prevention (AFSP), as well as suicide postvention teams through the VA. He also mentioned that more resources were being added to the chat by symposium participants.

Bruce Crow, who served as the VA's point of contact for the symposium planning committee, pointed to the importance of acknowledging the emotional impact of veteran suicide—something not normally considered a social determinant of health but that does impact the individual. This could be an approach that "broadens our thinking about what constitutes a social determinant," he commented.

BLACK VETERANS

The reporter for the group focusing on Black veterans stated that this group chose to focus on financial/employment problems. This was in part because this adverse social determinant of health acted as a "catch-all" for this population, he said. It reflects the more general findings that "African American veterans generally do well in every category compared to the African American community, but they still do worse when it comes to the veteran community." This is true of unemployment rates, with Black veterans having higher rates of unemployment and unemployability than the general veteran population, he noted. The reporter pointed to the Center for Minority Veterans report as the source of this observation. He also noted that underemployment contributes to financial/employment problems.

The reporter for the group emphasized that the lack of data on this population are a huge barrier to designing and implementing interventions. He noted that data exists, but it is scattered across institutions and "is just not in a place where we can . . . make really good scientific analysis."

The group highlighted systemic bias, especially in terms of access to benefits, as one aspect of financial/employment problems as an adverse social determinant of health for Black veterans. "How many African Americans who apply for benefits get denied?" This included support in the wake of military sexual trauma, the reporter noted.

Another challenge in this area discussed by the group was the lack of organizations that serve the Black veteran community, the reporter stated. He noted that there is often not proportional representation among stakeholders in these organizations. Of his own experience, the reporter commented, "Normally, I am the only African American in the room" alongside "White males, older, who are Republican." The reporter observed that this contrasts with the active duty population, which is more diverse. He also explained that in these contexts, race is often treated as a "divisive topic," which "really stops the conversation."

The reporter said the group considered that this lack of support for African American veterans may stem from a gap between Black legacy services (including the NAACP, the Urban League, the Congressional Black Caucus), which often "do not bring out the veteran issues," and veteran services, which often underserve Black veterans. The reporter mentioned the NAACP as one organization that does work at this intersection.

The group highlighted better data collection as a foundational part of any intervention that might address financial/employment problems, the group reporter said. "If I do not have the data, I cannot justify building a service." "We have to have more intersectional data," he commented in specific reference to Black women veterans and military sexual trauma.

Two strategies the group thought of to increase the store of data on this population included working with data already collected by the NAACP, and funding research at Historically Black Colleges and Universities. The reporter said the group also emphasized the importance of raising awareness around the work and needs of Black veterans. He suggested the creation of an award named after Alwyn Cashe, an African American recipient of the Medal of Honor; this award "would be presented every year to the veteran or a spouse of a veteran who did something for the community," the reporter said, as an effort to raise awareness.

WOMEN VETERANS

The reporter for this discussion group focused on women veterans stated that the topic they addressed was the importance social connection in the prevention of suicide among women veterans. The group created a "holistic transitional roadmap to civilian life" with the aim of providing "structure and navigational support to decrease the chance of personal crisis that could lead to suicide." The reporter emphasized the benefit of a holistic approach rather than focusing solely on career or another area of life, which research has shown leads to a feeling of unfulfillment. This is an upstream approach, she noted, including supporting transition before members leave active service.

This holistic approach covered four domains, the reporter for the group said: career and vocation; health (physical mental, emotional, relational, spiritual); relationships (family, friends, co-workers; "Who is in your support network beyond service?"); and time and money. The group emphasized the central role of collaboration and coalition-building, and partnering with existing organizations, in implementing this roadmap. "We want to collaborate between multiple entities to provide resources and support from military service through civilian life." This is "partnering on a grand scale," she noted, and might span the local, state, and federal levels.

The reporter for the group also reported the group's discussion regarding barriers to this intervention. One such challenge includes lack of access to service members on military bases. The EGS Sponsorship program would be a good partner "since they already have the seeds and groundwork on the bases." Marketing would also need to be "phrased appropriately" when communicating about collaboration between different service providers to people who might resist branching out. Training and staffing is also an important component of implementation, particularly in collaborative situations, she said. The participant also noted that measuring data and doing evaluation could present challenges when looking to create a holistic view of transition; one route might be through data from the VA's Personal Health Inventory, which is easily accessible and "asks all of these holistic questions." Devising surveys to study this question is also an option.

One purpose of this holistic roadmap would be to help give women service members transitioning out of active military service a plan that supports a sense of purpose and sense of clear vision for the future, the reporter noted, so that "hopefully [the veteran will] get pulled by the vision instead of getting pulled back by the pain or uncertainty or lack of clarity." The reporter also pointed to resources, including a mental health app from the VA that includes resources for military sexual trauma and PTSD.

8

Discussion of Interactive Session Reports and Synthesis of the Symposium

Strauman (Duke University) opened the general discussion of the breakout groups by highlighting some themes that came to the fore in the individual presentations. One such theme was "the importance of thinking about facilitating transitions for different groups." Another theme centered "getting local," or, "the importance of addressing social determinants at a very localized level" in part by empowering communities to do some of this work. A third theme was the use of "non-mental health professionals for suicide prevention." Among those mentioned were veteran service organizations, trained law enforcement personnel, and veteran peer mentorship programs, he noted. Related to the third theme was a fourth, the emphasis placed on the potential for suicide prevention "outside the clinical setting." The repeated call for more data on these subgroups—and not just more, but better, more accessible, more granular data collected not just as an afterthought—was the fifth and last theme highlighted by Strauman.

Strauman also added his own reflections on the material. Noting the "strong people" doing work in this area, he wondered how to incorporate the passion and commitment of individuals at the level of processes and programs so that when a strong person leaves, the organization or program continues to thrive. "How do we build . . . and sustain that enthusiasm and excitement and commitment and passion and bake it in as a process?" Strauman also emphasized the importance of acknowledging the different experiences, perspectives, and knowledge that each individual brings to collaborative and community work "so that we can work together to find that middle ground so that we can work collaboratively toward the solution."

CROSS-CUTTING THEMES ACROSS INTERACTIVE SESSIONS

Summarized below are cross-cutting themes among discussion groups that were identified during the full group discussion. These themes emerged in multiple discussion topics, and discussed in greater detail when the groups convened together.

Military Sexual Trauma

Discussion turned first to the association between MST and suicide. One symposium participant commented that it is not just an issue for women veterans; "three out of four sexual assaults that occur are actually male veterans." She suggested that advocacy by women veterans do stand to improve the situation for everyone affected. She also noted that the changing role of women veterans (in that women can be members of units that were previously not open to them) should be part of the larger discussion about MST. Moderator and committee member Rajeev Ramchand added that caring for the current cohort of veterans involves helping deal with the aftermath of MST in the past; and at the same time, "we prepare for the safety of future veterans." In this, he remarked, "it is so important for the DoD [Department of Defense] to be working on preventing MST and creating social environments that do not perpetuate MST." One participant noted that existing and new legislation that doesn't support women veterans even though they exist in high numbers and have a disproportionately high suicide rate, and "the main reason is military sexual trauma."

Evelyn Lewis observed that MST is "endemic throughout the military." She noted that 2021 had the "highest number of MSTs within the service academies that had ever been recorded since they've been collecting the data." Lewis also stressed the importance of approaching this problem with patient's perspective and also "the big picture" in mind: that is, other challenges that arise as a result of MST. She said MST is so traumatizing that it is an average of 12 years before the individual will begin to talk about it; this can result in the destruction of families, marriages, drugs abuse, homelessness: "All kinds of things just simply because they have not dealt with the initial MST experience and what it did to them." Another symposium participant pointed to the legal system as "the only way we are going to get rid of military sexual trauma" and referenced legislation passed by Texas in 2021 that moves the responsibility for investigating and prosecuting MST from military forces to law enforcement.

John Blosnich emphasized the necessity of having data in order to plan interventions. "Imagine if you are trying to plan an intervention for a group you cannot measure and in some cases were kind of disallowed to measure," he said. Blosnich also made a second point about social determinants of health often being at the root of "what we actually have to address within a health care system." He observed that adverse social determinants of health are "generating these social problems that come to a finer point for minority populations that we have to wrestle with." Blosnich advocated for "very honest conversations about the politics that undergird some of the social problems we are looking at."

Cohort Effect

Ramchand reported that a symposium participant observed via chat that while historically, suicide risk has been highest for senior citizens, recent evidence shows an increase in rates among young people. The symposium participant wondered how to know if this higher prevalence is "cohort specific," and will remain associated with that cohort through their life course, increasing in older age. In response, Lewis commented that nationalized perspective can show something different than a state or community view. "Suicide is so personal; you just cannot nationalize it." She noted that while the national number shows an uptick in young people dying by suicide, in Florida—for example—it is "the older generation" who has the highest prevalence of death by suicide, compared with other age groups. "We miss that [when] we try to nationalize the problem and use that as a solution." Ramchand agreed, commenting that being careful when thinking about rates and numbers is perhaps the point. "The national data does suggest that the numbers of suicide are much higher among the older veterans nationally." But, he said, the rate of suicide among the younger age cohort has certainly increased.

Turning back to the question of whether this is a cohort effect, Strauman said that he did not know, but offered two ways of looking at it. Looking at international data shows "the same basic trend"—a "sort of depths of despair phenomenon" visible in the United States and internationally. But, he noted, it is also reasonable to think that it may not be "simply a cohort effect, because the kind of risk factors we have been talking about predict this increase in suicide rates, particularly in younger and middle-aged people across these different countries." He acknowledged that this big picture perspective "overlooks a whole lot of variability that is regional and cultural and personal," but looking at the increase from this perspective does seem to indicate that "the variability in these predictors" may be behind it. Strauman noted that this increase in suicide rates among younger people was one impetus for the symposium itself and the posing of these kinds of questions. "We have to do it at multiple levels," he noted. It is important not to lose sight of the fact that suicide is about "one person at a time," and also use regional, national, and international data in the work of understanding what is driving this increase.

The Impact of a Long War

Building on the conversation about a cohort effect being behind the increase in suicide rates among young people, a symposium participant pointed to the possible impacts of an "elongated war." He noted that the present war is not defined in the same way as earlier wars, which have a defined starting point and an ending point, and neither does it fit in between these wars the way other conflicts, such as the Cold War or the "post-Desert Shield/Desert Storm" eras. In this case, he noted, "we still have people in Iraq. We still have people in Bosnia. We still have people in different places [and] we still do not understand what it is doing to them." He noted that three words sometimes associated with World War 2 veterans are honor, courage, and dignity. By contrast, words associated with a veteran of Iraq or Afghanistan might be "broken," "PTSD," and other negative words.

Suicide as a Manifestation of Societal Stress, Businesses as Potential Collaborative Partners

One important domain to look into is "suicide as a manifestation of societal stress" in the same way that "domestic violence, substance abuse, [and] child abuse" are, said an symposium participant. He reiterated the importance of connecting veterans with resources, especially but not only before and during separation. He drew attention to companies as potential partners, and pointed to Optum Serve, a program by Optum at the United Health Group, which he represented, as an example. Optum Serve supports veterans in this way and has a strong peer support system with "a number of virtual and interactive platforms," he said. He urged listeners to look into what such businesses might offer, as they look for collaborative partners and build coalitions.

Incarcerated Veterans

A symposium participant raised the importance of research around incarcerated veterans. He mentioned that in his home area of Southern Nevada, over the past three years, there has been an increase in veterans being incarcerated; upon release, he said, an increased percentage has become homeless or "lost in the shuffle." Ramchand noted that one place to look at this intersection between the veterans in the criminal justice system and suicide risk might be through the medical-legal partnerships at the VA and elsewhere. He also mentioned a group of researchers looking at suicide prevention in criminal justice settings, but noted that this is different than this point of release is also "another point of transition" where "some veterans could be at risk, doubly at risk" perhaps.

SYNTHESIS OF THE SYMPOSIUM

Strauman concluded the symposium with a synthesis of the sessions. He began by highlighting several terms that capture what he saw as key themes. The first of these terms was "holistic," which highlights the idea that an individual's needs "cannot be put into a single category" and addressed only within that limited scope. This points to the importance of seeing that "suicide prevention is something that benefits people in other ways and other kinds of interventions have suicide preventive value."

Strauman's second highlighted term was "individualized," which pointed to the importance of designing suicide prevention measures that are "in a modality that makes [the targeted] people comfortable as individuals." He pointed to the many discussions in the symposium about intersectionality, including identities, communities, people's histories, cohort effects, and individual experience. Third, Strauman highlighted the concept of "ceding power to individuals and communities," a phrase borrowed from an audience participant. Fourth on Strauman's list was how "urgent" the problem of MST is, as seen in part through the data coming out of service academies, as mentioned in the group discussion by Lewis. "It is something that people I think at the national level may not be comfortable talking about, but it is a conversation that has to occur," he said.

The fifth term Strauman included in his synthesis was "logistics," meaning "how do we get the resources that people need to them." This might include "everything from broadband to trucks" as well as help connecting to services and resources; and such work must be done at all levels, he commented, including "individual community meetings" as well as "virtual, online, national conferences, and academies." "Politics" was the sixth and last term Strauman mentioned, calling it "an elephant in the room." He commented, "some of these topics are not going to be [politically] popular, and yet we owe it to our veteran population to be as courageous and open as we can about it in these discussions."

Ramchand continued the synthesis by highlighting the conversation around the need for more, better quality, and more timely data. He reflected, "It was really encouraging to hear you all talk about how you also prioritize the need for data to help you strengthen your programs and your intervention efforts, [and] your evaluation efforts." Ramchand also pointed to a theme throughout the symposium around "thinking outside the box," that is, thinking how suicide prevention might be done outside of the clinical setting as well as in it. He praised the work being done by clinicians in the bio-medical field, but noted "it is a limited supply out there who are doing that work." Expanding beyond this group is important as need expands, he said.

Lewis echoed the call for more and better data, and also reminded the group that behind the data are real people. "As we conduct the research and collect this data, the people impacted by these issues are waiting on us, relying on us, depending on us to come back to the table with solutions to the issues that impact their lives on a daily basis." She noted that "it is incumbent upon us to get this right now," meaning, to get data that will "have the greatest impact on the lives of those who are in need of answers."

Bruce Crow, who served as the VA's point of contact for the symposium planning committee, expressed his appreciation for the work done by the National Academies, particularly the Planning Committee, for putting together the symposium. He noted that he is coming away from the symposium "with a sense of optimism, looking at the people who are involved, the perspectives, the commitment, the passion [for] preventing veteran suicide, the level of interest." He expressed "great hope that we are indeed going to make a difference."

References

Blosnich, J., Montgomery, A., Dichter, M.E., Gordon, A.J., Kavalieratos, D., Taylor, L., Ketterer, B., & Bossarte, R.M. (2019). Social determinants and military veterans' suicide ideation and attempt: A cross-sectional analysis of electronic health record data. *Journal of General Internal Medicine, 35,* 1759–1767.

Boston: 3-D Commission. (2021). *Data, Social Determinants, and Better Decision-Making for Health: The Report of the 3-D Commission.* https://static1.squarespace.com/static/5e2ca08b9fdf240fb1abb55b/t/617aae3927d4790b590aef4e/1635429947691/3D Commission_Report_SDoH_Oct+12_final.pdf.

Bowman, P.J. (2006). Role strain and adaptation issues in the strength-based model: Diversity, multilevel, and life-span considerations. *The Counseling Psychologist, 34*(1), 120.

Boyer, T.L., Youk, A.O., Haas, A.P., Brown, G.R., Shipherd, J.C., Kauth, M.R., Jasuja, G.K., & Blosnich, J.R. (2021). Suicide, homicide, and all-cause mortality among transgender and cisgender patients in the Veterans Health Administration. *LGBT Health, 8*(3), 173–180.

Branas, C.C., Kondo, M.C., Murphy, S.M., South, E.C., Polsky, D., & MacDonald, J.M. (2016). Urban blight remediation as a cost-beneficial solution to firearm violence. *American Journal of Public Health, 106*(12), 2158–2164.

Branas, C.C., South, E., Kondo, M.C., Hohl, B.C., Bourgois, P., Wiebe, D.J., & MacDonald, J.M. (2018). A citywide cluster randomized trial to restore blighted vacant land and its effects on violence, crime and fear. *Proceedings of the National Academy of Sciences, 115*(8), 1–11.

Bridge, J.A., Horowitz, L.M., Fontanella, C.A., et al. (2018). Age-related racial disparity in suicide rates among U.S. youths from 2001 through 2015. *Journal of American Medicine: Pediatrics, 172*(7), 697.

Bullman, T., Hoffmire, C., Schneiderman, A., & Bossarte, R. (2015). Time dependent gender differences in suicide risk among Operation Enduring Freedom and Operation Iraqi Freedom veterans. *Annals of Epidemiology, 25*(12), 964–965. doi: https://doi.org/10.1016/j.annepidem.2015.09.008.

Centers for Disease Control and Prevention (CDC). (2016). *Behavior Risk Factor Surveillance System*. https://www.cdc.gov/brfss/index.html.

Centers for Disease Control and Prevention. (2017). *Web-Based Injury Statistics Query and Reporting System*. https://www.cdc.gov/injury/wisqars/index.html.

Centers for Disease Control and Prevention. (2017). *"Preventing Suicide: A Technical Package of Policy, Programs, and Practices."* National Center for Injury Prevention and Control. Atlanta, GA: Author. https://www.cdc.gov/violenceprevention/pdf/suicidetechnicalpackage.pdf.

Collarbone, P. (2009). *Creating Tomorrow: Planning, Developing, and Sustaining Change in Education and Other Public Services*. London: Bloomsbury.

Culhane, D., Szymkowiak, D., & Schinka, J.A. (2019). Suicidality and the onset of homelessness: Evidence for a temporal association from VHA treatment records. *Psychiatric Services, 70*(11), 1049–1052.

Davydenko, M., Kolbuszewska, M., & Peetz, J. (2021). A meta-analysis of financial self-control strategies: Comparing empirical findings with online media and lay person perspectives on what helps individuals curb spending and start saving. *PLoS One, 16*(7), e0253938.

de la Garza, Á.G., Blanco, C., Olfson, M., & Wall, M.M. (2021). Identification of suicide attempt risk factors in a national US survey using machine learning. *JAMA Psychiatry, 78*(4), 398–406.

Elbogen, E.B., Molloy, K., Wagner, H.R., Kimbrel, N., Beckham, J.C., Van Male, L., Leinbach, J., & Bradford, D.W. (2020a). Psychosocial protective factors and suicidal ideation: Results from a National Longitudinal Study of Veterans. *Journal of Affective Disorders, 260*, 703–709.

Elbogen, E.B., Lanier, M., Montgomery, A.E., Strickland, S., Wagner, H.R., & Tsai, J. (2020b). Financial strain and suicide attempts in a nationally representative sample of U.S. adults. *American Journal of Epidemiology, 189*, 1266–1274.

Gellar, E.S. (2008). People-based leadership enriching a work culture for world-class safety. *Professional Safety, 53*(3), 29–36.

Hoffberg, A.S., Spitzer, E., Mackelprang, J.L., Farro, S.A., & Brenner, L.A. (2018). Suicidal self-directed violence among homeless U.S. veterans: A systematic review. *Suicide and Life-Threatening Behavior, 48*(4), 481–498.

Hoffmire, C.A., Borowski, S., Griffin, B.J., Maguen, S., & Vogt, D. (2022). Trajectories of suicidal ideation following separation from military service: Overall trends and group differences. *Suicide & Life-Threatening Behavior*. Advance online publication. doi: https://doi.org/10.1111/sltb.12831.

Hoffmire, C.A., Monteith, L.M., Forster, J.E., Bernhard, P.A., Blosnich, J.R., Vogt, D., Maguen, S., Smith, A.A., & Schneiderman, A.I. (2021). Gender differences in lifetime prevalence and onset timing of suicidal ideation and suicide attempt among post-9/11 veterans and nonveterans. *Medical Care, 59*, S84–S91. https://doi.org/10.1097/mlr.0000000000001431.

Hottes, T.S., Bogaert, L., Rhodes, A.E., Brennan, D.J., & Gesink, D. (2016). Lifetime prevalence of suicide attempts among sexual minority adults by study sampling strategies: A systematic review and meta-analysis. *American Journal of Public Health, 106*(5), e1–e12. doi: 10.2105/AJPH.2016.303088.

Indian Health Service. (2019). *Indian Health Disparities*. https://www.ihs.gov/newsroom/factsheets/disparities/.

Ivey-Stephenson, A.Z., Crosby, A.E., Jack, S.P.D., Haileyesus, T., & Kresnow-Sedacca, M.J. (2017). Suicide trends among and within urbanization levels by sex, race/ethnicity, age group, and mechanism of death—United States, 2001–2015. *MMWR Surveillance Summaries, 66*(18), 1–16.

Jackson, J.S., Torres, M., Caldwell, C.H., Neighbors, H.W. Nesse, R.M., Taylor, R.J., Trierweiler S.J., & Williams, D.R. (2004). The National Survey of American Life: A study of racial, ethnic and cultural influences on mental disorders and mental health. *International Journal of Methods in Psychiatric Research*, 13(4), 196–207. doi: 10.1002/mpr.177.

Jones, J.M. (2021). *LGBT Identification Rises to 5.6% in Latest U.S. Estimate*. Gallup. https://news.gallup.com/poll/329708/lgbt-identification-rises-latest-estimate.aspx.

Mashek, D. (2015, June). *Capacities and Institutional Supported Needed Along the Collaboration Continuum*. A presentation to the Academic Deans Committee of The Claremont Colleges, Claremont. CA.

Melnyk, B.M. (2020). Reducing healthcare costs for mental health hospitalizations with the evidence-based COPE program for child and adolescent depression and anxiety: A cost analysis. *Journal of Pediatric Health Care*, 34(2), 117–121. doi: 10.1016/j.pedhc.2019.08.002.

Mohatt, N.V., Hoffmire, C.A., Schneider, A.L.B., Goss, C.W., Shore, J.H., Spark, T.L., & Kaufman, C.E. (2022). Suicide among American Indian and Alaska Native veterans who use Veterans Health Administration care. *Medical Care*, 60(4), 275–278 doi: 10.1097/MLR.0000000000001656.

Mohatt, N.V., Kreisel, C.J., Hoffberg, A.S., Wendleton, L., & Beehler, S.J. (2020). A systematic review of factors impacting suicide risk among rural adults in the United States. *The Journal of Rural Health*. Advanced online publication. doi: 10.1111/jrh.12532.

Monteith, L.L., Holliday, R., Miller, C., Schneider, A.L., Hoffmire, C.A., Bahraini, N.H., & Forster, J.E. (2020). Suicidal ideation, suicide attempt, and non-suicidal self-injury among female veterans: prevalence, timing, and onset. *Journal of Affective Disorders*, 273, 350–357. https://doi.org/10.1016/j.jad.2020.04.017.

Moyer, R., MacDonald, J., Ridgeway, G., & Branas, C. (2019). Effect of remediating blighted vacant land on shootings: A citywide cluster randomized trial. *American Public Health Association*, 109(1), 140–144. https://doi.org/10.2105/AJPH.2018.304752.

National Academies of Sciences, Engineering, and Medicine (NASEM). (2021). *High and Rising Mortality Rates Among Working-Age Adults*. Washington, DC: The National Academies Press. https://doi.org/10.17226/25976.

Nelson, R.E., Montgomery, A.E., Suo, Y., Cook, J., Pettey, W., Gundlapalli, A., Greene, T., Evans, W., Gelberg, L., Kertesz, S.G., Tsai, J., & Byrne, T.H. (2021). Temporary financial assistance decreased health care costs for veterans experiencing housing instability. *Health Affairs*, 40(5), 820–828.

Richardson, T., Elliott, P., & Roberts, R. (2013). The relationship between personal unsecured debt and mental and physical health: A systematic review and meta-analysis. *Clinical Psychology Review*, 33(8), 1148–1162. doi: 10.1016/j.cpr.2013.08.009.

Roser, M. (2017). Link between health spending and life expectancy: The U.S. is an outlier. *Our World in Data*. https://ourworldindata.org/the-link-between-life-expectancy-and-health-spending-us-focus.

Russell, S.T., Pollitt, A.M., Li, G., & Grossman, A.H. (2018). Chosen name use is linked to reduced depressive symptoms, suicidal ideation, and suicidal behavior among transgender youth. *Journal of Adolescent Health*, 63(4), 503–505.

Tsai, J., & Cao, X. (2019). Association between suicide attempts and homelessness in a population-based sample of US veterans and non-veterans. *Journal of Epidemiology and Community Health*, 73(4), 346–352.

Vogt, D., Taverna, E.C., Nillni, Y.I., Booth, B., Perkins, D.F., Copeland, L.A., Finley, E.P., Tyrell, F.A., & Gilman, C.L. (2019). Development and validation of a tool to assess military veterans' status, functioning, and satisfaction with key aspects of their lives. *Applied Psychology. Health and Well-Being*, 11(2), 328–349. https://doi.org/10.1111/aphw.12161.

Appendix A

Symposium Agenda

Community Interventions to Prevent Veteran Suicide:
The Role of Social Determinants
A Symposium

March 28–29, 2022
Time EDT

SYMPOSIUM OBJECTIVES

To gain a better understanding of social determinants influencing the recent increase in suicide risk and how currently available practice guidelines can inform community-level preventive interventions, particularly those targeting veteran populations. The symposium will address: the relevant social, cultural, and economic factors driving changes in suicide risk among veterans (1) and ways that current best practices for suicide prevention and treatment can be applied at the community level (2).

DAY ONE

11:00 Welcoming Remarks from DBASSE and Introductions

Samantha Chao, Board on Behavioral, Cognitive, and Sensory Sciences. Division of Behavioral and Social Sciences and Education (DBASSE)

11:10 Welcoming Remarks from the Sponsor

Matthew Miller, Executive Director of VA Suicide Prevention, Department of Veterans Affairs

11:20 Overview of Meeting Agenda and Framing the Symposium

Timothy Strauman, Committee Chair, Duke University

Session One: Overview and Understanding of the Evidence on Social, Cultural, and Economic Determinants Related to Suicide

In this session speakers will:
- define terms (e.g., social determinants of health [SDOH]; risk and protective factors for suicide; etc.)
- summarize the evidence on the social, cultural, and economic factors related to suicide in the general population, and among veterans
- provide a common ground understanding of factors that contribute to suicide among veterans at individual (micro) and system/societal (macro) levels
- summarize research on the particular influences of social, cultural, and economic determinants of suicide and other health-related outcomes on unique groups of people; and discuss the implication for interventions

Committee Moderator: Debra Houry, CDC

11:30 Sandro Galea (NAM), Boston University – *Overview of social determinants of health (SDOH)*

11:45 Eric Elbogen, Duke University; VA National Center on Homelessness Among Veterans – *Financial distress and suicide*

12:00 Irma Elo, University of Pennsylvania – *Trends, disparities, and explanations for suicide mortality among working age adults*

12:15 Q & A

APPENDIX A 79

Committee Moderator: Evelyn Lewis, Retired Navy, Veterans Health and Wellness Foundation

12:30 Nathaniel Mohatt, VA RMIRECC and University of Colorado – *SDOH and suicide/other health outcomes among rural populations*

12:45 **Pamela End of Horn,** Indian Health Service – *SDOH and suicide/other health outcomes among American Indian/Native Alaska populations*

1:00 Claire Hoffmire, VA Office of Mental Health and Suicide Prevention – *SDOH and suicide/other health outcomes among women*

1:15 Q & A

1:30 LUNCH BREAK

Committee Moderator: Rajeev Ramchand, Rand

2:15 John Blosnich, University of Southern California – *SDOH and suicide/other health outcomes among LGBTQ+ populations*

2:30 Kim Van Orden, University of Rochester Medical Center – *SDOH and suicide/other health outcomes among elderly populations*

2:45 Sean Joe, Washington University in St. Louis – *Dual trends of increasing suicide rates among Black youth and projected increases of Black/African American veterans*

3:00 Q & A

Session Two: Community Interventions to Address
Social, Cultural, and Economic Determinants

This session will have two panels focusing on community interventions and elements of community interventions and coalitions that have been used to prevent suicide and other health outcomes.

Topics to be covered:
- What social, cultural, and economic determinants of health does the community intervention address? How are these measured?
- What are the public health outcomes targeted for change/impact?

- What are the main program components of the community intervention?
- Are "coalitions/community partnerships/ collaborations" a primary component of the community intervention?
- What are the key elements of the "coalitions/community partnerships/collaborations"? How are these measured?
- How is measurement used to assess program implementation, progress, and outcomes?
- What is the evidence base for the community intervention? Have population outcomes been measured?
- What guidance/ideas about competencies and strategies could be offered, as well as blueprints for developing community interventions?

PANEL A. Community Interventions for Suicide Prevention and Support for Veterans
Committee Moderator: Lisa Brenner, University of Colorado; MIRECC

3:15   VA GOVERNOR'S CHALLENGE INITIATIVE ON SUICIDE PREVENTION – Nicola Winkel, Arizona Governor's Challenge and Arizona Coalition for Military Families

3:30   LETHAL MEANS SAFETY – Joseph Simonetti, Rocky Mountain Regional VA Medical Center; University of Colorado

3:45   CDC "PREVENTING SUICIDE: A TECHNICAL PACKAGE OF POLICIES, PROGRAMS, AND PRACTICES" – Debra Houry (NAM) Centers for Disease Control and Prevention

4:00   Q & A

PANEL B. Community Interventions for Varied Applications in Housing, Health, and Safety
Committee Moderator: Tim Strauman, Chair, Duke University

4:30   SUPPORTIVE SERVICES FOR VETERAN FAMILIES – Jack Tsai, University of Texas, Houston; Veterans Health Administration, Homeless Programs Office

4:45   FROM NETWORKS TO COLLECTIVE IMPACT: WHICH FORM OF COLLABORATION IS BEST FOR YOU? – Holly Raffle, Ohio University

Community level interventions to address social determinants of health are built on interorganizational networks that link people, neighborhoods, communities, and public and private organizations in design, implementation, and evaluation. This presentation will highlight various forms of such collaboration as well as their characteristics, requirements, and processes.

5:00 PLACE-BASED INTERVENTIONS TO ADDRESS VACANCY AND ABANDONMENT – Charles Branas (NAM), Mailman School of Public Health, Columbia University
Theory, evidence, and examples of place-based interventions to improve environments and help create safe and healthy neighborhoods.

5:15 Q & A

5:30 Wrap Up for Day 1; Charge for Day 2
Timothy Strauman

5:35 Adjourn Day One

DAY TWO

11:00 Opening Remarks and Overview of Day Two
Timothy Strauman, Duke University

11:10 Introduction to Breakout Exercises and Getting Set up in Zoom Breakout Rooms
Molly Dorries and Ashton Bullock, Board on Behavioral, Cognitive, and Sensory Sciences

11:30 Interactive Breakout Sessions
Participants will be divided into breakout groups. The task of each group is to apply information gained from the first day of the symposium to processes of designing, implementing, and evaluating community interventions.

1:00 LUNCH BREAK

1:45 Reports and Discussion from Breakout Groups
Rajeev Ramchand, RAND

3:15 BREAK

3:30 Synthesis of Symposium Sessions
      Timothy Strauman and Committee

4:00 Adjourn Symposium

Appendix B

Biographical Sketches of Planning Committee Members and Presenters

PLANNING COMMITTEE MEMBERS

Timothy J. Strauman *(Chair)*, Ph.D., is a professor and former chair of the Department of Psychology and Neuroscience at Duke University and also professor of psychiatry and behavioral sciences in the Duke University School of Medicine. His research interests focus on the psychological and neurobiological processes of self-regulation, conceptualized in terms of a cognitive/motivational perspective, as well as on the relation between self-regulation and affect and how such processes might contribute to psychopathology. His lab's clinically focused research includes the development and validation of a new self-regulation-based therapy for depression, self-system therapy, and the use of neuroimaging techniques to examine the mechanisms of action of treatments for depression. He is a former president of the Academy of Psychological Clinical Science, a fellow of the Association for Psychological Science, a current member of the Board on Behavioral, Cognitive, and Sensory Sciences, and a founding fellow of the Academy of Cognitive Therapy. He has a Ph.D. in clinical psychology from New York University.

Lisa A. Brenner, Ph.D., is a board-certified rehabilitation psychologist, a professor of Physical Medicine and Rehabilitation (PM&R), Psychiatry, and Neurology at the University of Colorado, as well as Anschutz Medical Campus, and the Director of the Department of Veterans Affairs Rocky Mountain Mental Illness Research, Education, and Clinical Center (MIRECC). She is also Vice Chair of Research for the Department of

PM&R. Brenner is the Past President of Division 22 (Rehabilitation Psychology) of the American Psychological Association (APA) and an APA Fellow. She serves as an Associate Editor of the Journal of Head Trauma Rehabilitation. Her primary area of research interest is traumatic brain injury, co-morbid psychiatric disorders, and negative psychiatric outcomes including suicide. Brenner has numerous peer-reviewed publications, participates on national advisory boards, and has recently co-authored a book titled: *Suicide Prevention After Neurodisability: An Evidence-Informed Approach.*

Mitzi Fields, M.S.N., is a Colonel in the U.S. Army and is currently serving as the deputy commanding officer/deputy commander for nursing at Fort Bliss in Texas.

Debra Houry, M.D., M.P.H., is the acting principal deputy director of Centers for Disease Control and Prevention (CDC). Since 2014, Houry served as director of the National Center for Injury Prevention and Control (NCIPC) at CDC. In this role, she led innovative research and science-based programs to prevent injuries and violence and to reduce their consequences. While at NCIPC, she oversaw the development of comprehensive suicide prevention program at CDC. Houry previously served as vice chair and associate professor in the Department of Emergency Medicine at Emory University School of Medicine and as associate professor at the Rollins School of Public Health. Houry has participated on numerous public health boards and committees. She has authored more than 100 peer-reviewed publications and book chapters, is a member of the National Academy of Medicine, and has received numerous awards throughout her career including the APHA Jay Drotman award. Houry received her M.D. and M.P.H. degrees from Tulane University and completed her residency training in emergency medicine at Denver Health Medical Center.

Evelyn L. Lewis, M.D., M.A., F.A.A.F.P., retired from the Navy after 25 years of service and currently serves as president and chairman Veterans Health and Wellness Foundation. She is nationally recognized for her expertise in the areas of Veteran health and health care issues; cultural competency; health and health care disparities and was recently selected to serve as a Senior Scientist/Investigator for the American Academy Family Physicians' National Research Network. Lewis earned her M.D. from the University of the Health Sciences, the Chicago Medical School and completed a residency in family medicine at Naval Hospital Jacksonville, Jacksonville, FL.

Rajeev Ramchand, Ph.D., is co-director of the RAND Epstein Family Veterans Policy Research Institute and a senior behavioral scientist at the

RAND Corporation. He studies the prevalence, prevention, and treatment of mental health and substance use disorders in adolescents, service members and veterans, and minority populations. He has conducted many studies on suicide and suicide prevention including environmental scans of suicide prevention programs, epidemiologic studies on risk factors for suicide, qualitative research with suicide loss survivors, and evaluations of suicide prevention programs. He has also developed freely available tools to help organizations to evaluate their own suicide prevention programs. He has testified on suicide prevention before the U.S. Senate, House of Representatives, and California State Senate. Other current areas of research include military and veteran caregivers; the role of firearm availability, storage, and policies on suicide; the impact of disasters on community health; and using public health approaches to study and prevent hate and violent extremism.

SYMPOSIUM SPEAKERS

John R. Blosnich, Ph.D., M.P.H., is an assistant professor at the Suzanne Dworak-Peck School of Social Work at the University of Southern California where his research focuses on health equity for lesbian, gay, bisexual, and transgender (LGBT) individuals, with a specific emphasis on social determinants of health and suicide risk. He has worked for 10 years with the VA, first with the Veterans Integrated Service Networks Center of Excellence for Suicide Prevention and then with the Center for Health Equity Research and Promotion at the VA Pittsburgh Healthcare System, where he pioneered research about LGBT veterans. Blosnich has garnered several research awards from both the VA and the National Institutes of Health. Most recently, Blosnich was a 2021 recipient of an National Institutes of Health Director's New Innovator Award, which supports his efforts to explore how to expand suicide prevention into nonclinical sectors in which adverse social factors and acute life crises can be targeted for upstream prevention.

Charles Branas, Ph.D., is a professor who directs the Department of Epidemiology and a CDC Research Center at Columbia University. His research extends from urban and rural areas in the United States to communities across the globe, incorporating place-based interventions and human geography. He has led science that generates new knowledge while simultaneously creating positive, real-world changes and health-enhancing resources with local communities. He has worked in multiple Schools of Public Health, Engineering, and Medicine, and is a member of the National Academy of Medicine.

Eric Elbogen, Ph.D., is a research investigator at the National Center on Homelessness Among Veterans and is professor in the Department of Psychiatry and Behavioral Sciences at the Duke University School of Medicine. He ran a money management group at the Durham VA for more than a decade and has been Principal Investigator of a randomized clinical trial of a recovery-oriented money management intervention for Veterans and of a nationally representative longitudinal survey of Veterans identifying a link between financial strain and suicidal ideation. Elbogen and colleagues also demonstrated a link between financial strain and suicide risk in the U.S. general population and during the COVID-19 pandemic.

Irma Elo, Ph.D., earned her Ph.D. in Demography and Public Affairs from Princeton University. She is the chair of the Sociology Department and a research associate at the Population Studies Center and the Population Aging Research Center at the University of Pennsylvania. She has served as a member and/or a chair of several national and international committees, including chair of the Board of Scientific Counselors of the National Center for Health Statistics, member of the Census Bureau's Scientific Advisory Committee, member and chair of the section on the sociology of population for the American Sociological Association, member of the Population Association of America's (PAA) board of directors, chair of the PAA's Committee on Population Statistics, and a member of an International Advisory Board of the Swedish Initiative for Research on Microdata in the Social and Medical Sciences. Her main research interests center on socioeconomic and racial/ethnic disparities in health, cognition, and mortality across the life course and demographic estimation of mortality. In recent years, she has extended this focus to include health and mortality among racial/ethnic immigrant subgroups. She is currently the principal investigator of National Institute on Aging-funded study, Causes of Geographic Divergence in U.S. Mortality.

Pamela End of Horn is a licensed independent clinical social worker in North Dakota and Minnesota. She focuses on Mental Health, specifically Suicide Prevention. End of Horn has worked in Suicide Prevention since 2007 within the Department of Veterans Affairs and Indian Health Service, and her primary goal is to continue working within Suicide Prevention in the American Indian population.

Sandro Galea, M.D., M.P.H., Dr.P.H., is a physician, epidemiologist, and author, is dean and Robert A. Knox Professor at Boston University School of Public Health. He previously held academic and leadership positions at Columbia University, the University of Michigan, and the New York Academy of Medicine. He has published extensively in the peer-reviewed literature, and is a regular contributor to a range of public media, about the social causes of health, mental health, and the consequences of trauma.

He has been listed as one of the most widely cited scholars in the social sciences. He is past chair of the board of the Association of Schools and Programs of Public Health and past president of the Society for Epidemiologic Research and of the Interdisciplinary Association for Population Health Science. He is an elected member of the National Academy of Medicine. Galea has received several lifetime achievement awards. Galea holds a medical degree from the University of Toronto, graduate degrees from Harvard University and Columbia University, and an honorary doctorate from the University of Glasgow.

Claire A. Hoffmire, Ph.D., serves as a principal investigator and co-lead for the ASPIRE Lab at the Department of Veterans Affairs Rocky Mountain Mental Illness Research Education and Clinical Center (MIRECC) for Veteran Suicide Prevention and Assistant Professor of Physical Medicine and Rehabilitation at the University of Colorado School of Medicine. Hoffmire is an Epidemiologist and has worked in the field of Veteran suicide prevention since 2012; her research aims to inform evidence-based suicide prevention programs for all Veterans, within and outside the VA. Hoffmire is committed to conducting research which can be leveraged to improve upstream, public-health oriented suicide prevention programs for historically underrepresented and underserved Veterans, such as women Veterans and Veterans not engaged in VA health care.

Debra Houry – see Committee Biographies

Sean Joe, Ph.D., is a nationally recognized scholar on suicidal behavior among Black Americans, particularly regarding the role of firearms as a risk factor, and is expanding the evidence base for effective practice with Black boys and young men. His research focuses on Black adolescents' mental health service use patterns, and father-focus family-based interventions to prevent urban Black American adolescent males from engaging in multiple forms of self-destructive behaviors. Joe is the president of the Society for Social Work and Research (SSWR), whose members represent more than 200 universities and institutions, 45 states in the United States as well as from 15 countries. SSWR advances, disseminates, and translates research that addresses issues of social work practice and policy and promotes a diverse, just, and equitable society. Joe is a Fellow of the American Academy of Social Work and Social Welfare, the Society for Social Work and Research, and New York Academy of Medicine. He serves on the Steering Committee of the national Suicide Prevention Resource Center, Standards, Training and Practices Committee of the National Suicide Prevention Lifeline, and the Scientific Advisory Board of the American Foundation for Suicide Prevention.

As founding director of the Race and Opportunity Lab, which examines race, opportunity, and social mobility with an emphasis on informing policies, interventions, and intra-professional practice to lessen ethnic inequality in adolescents' healthy transition to adulthood. The lab leading community science project is HomeGrown STL, which is a multi-systemic placed-based capacity building intervention to enhance upward mobility opportunities and health of Black males ages 12-29 years in the St. Louis region. His epistemological work focuses on the concept of race in medical and social sciences.

Nathaniel Mohatt, Ph.D., is a community psychologist and leader of community-based suicide prevention programs within the U.S. Department of Veterans Affairs. He is Principal Investigator and Program Lead of the VA's Together with Veterans Rural Suicide Prevention Program and serves as a consultant for Community-Based Suicide Prevention to the VA's National Office of Mental Health and Suicide Prevention. Mohatt holds appointments as an Assistant Professor of Physical Medicine and Rehabilitation at the University of Colorado Anschutz Medical Campus and as a Research Psychologist with the VA Rocky Mountain Mental Illness Research, Education, and Clinical Center. In his research, he employs community based participatory research and health equity frameworks to develop and implement effective and culturally responsive prevention programs and health care services for rural and indigenous populations.

Holly Raffle, Ph.D., professor of Leadership and Public Affairs, leads the Partnership for Community-Based Prevention (P4CBP) at Ohio University's Voinovich School of Leadership and Public Affairs. As an engaged faculty, she is responsible for leading a portfolio of work centered on community-based behavioral health, focusing on promotion and prevention efforts. Since 2009, the P4CBP has generated nearly $20 million in external funding from partner organizations such as the Ohio Department of Mental Health and Addiction Services (OhioMHAS), the U.S. Health Resources & Services Administration, the Substance Abuse and Mental Health Services Administration and 22 other sponsors. During that timeframe, the P4CBP has collaborated to provide intensive leadership development, training, technical assistance, implementation support, workforce development, and evaluation services to 84 Ohio communities as they address critical needs and issues related to mental health and substance use disorder. In 2021, OhioMHAS officially named the Voinovich School as the home of the Ohio Center of Excellence for Behavioral Health Prevention and Promotion; Raffle is honored to serve as the founding Faculty Director. Raffle was the recipient of the 2013 Firefly Award from the Fairfield County Family, Adult, and Children First Council recognizing her commitment to community-level prevention. Raffle was the recipient of the 2014 OhioMHAS Prevention Champion

Award, recognizing her efforts to support state agencies, Behavioral Health Boards, and prevention providers rethink or redesign their prevention systems through the Strategic Prevention Framework. Additionally, she is a Master Certified Health Education Specialist an active member of the Society for Public Health Education (SOPHE) as well as the Ohio SOPHE, where she served a three-year term on the Board of Directors.

Joseph Simonetti, M.D., M.P.H., earned his M.D. from The Ohio State University in 2008 and trained in Internal Medicine at the University of Pittsburgh. He then completed an NRSA health services research fellowship, worked as a senior research fellow at the Harborview Injury Prevention & Research Center at the University of Washington and the VA's Patient Aligned Care Team National Demonstration Lab, and earned his M.P.H. from the University of Washington School of Public Health. Currently, he is a physician practicing within the VA Eastern Colorado Healthcare System, whose research focuses on reducing the burden of intentional and unintentional firearm injuries nationally. Within VA, his focus is on creating infrastructure for stakeholder engagement in firearm-related research and developing Veteran-centered approaches to facilitating lethal means safety as a suicide prevention strategy.

Jack Tsai, Ph.D., serves as campus dean and professor of public health at the University of Texas Health Science Center at Houston. He previously served on faculty at Yale School of Medicine where he directed the Division of Mental Health Services. He has received federally funded grants and published more than 200 peer-reviewed studies on homelessness, severe mental illness, trauma, and health disparities. He has held elected leadership positions in the American Psychological Association and the American Public Health Association, and also serves as Editor-in-Chief for *Mental Health Research* and the *Journal of Social Distress and Homelessness*.

Kimberly Van Orden, Ph.D., is a clinical psychologist and associate professor in the Department of Psychiatry at the University of Rochester Medical Center (URMC). She directs the HOPE Lab (Helping Older People Engage), which studies programs to promote social connection and healthy aging and prevent suicide in later life. She co-directs the Rochester Roybal Center for Social Ties and Aging, which is focused on promoting social vitality for dementia family caregivers. She co-directs the Center for the Study and Prevention of Suicide at URMC, as well as a research fellowship in suicide prevention. She mentors students and fellows and maintains a clinical practice providing evidence-based psychotherapy to older adults.

Nicola Winkel, M.P.A., is project director, Arizona Coalition for Military Families. She specializes in program development and implementation, bringing a mix of planning, project management, communication, team coordination and problem solving skills that drive execution of complex projects and build sustainability. Winkel has worked for more than 20 years in the nonprofit community, including a lead development and implementation role in the creation and growth of the Arizona Coalition for Military Families, a nationally-recognized public/private partnership focused on building Arizona's capacity to care for and support all service members, veterans, their families and communities. She has also had a principal role in the development and implementation of Arizona's Be Connected program, which focuses on upstream prevention to positively impact social determinants of health and decrease the risk of suicide. In addition to her work with the Coalition, Ms. Winkel has provided consulting services for state and national initiatives, including the Be Resilient Program with the Arizona National Guard; Continuing education programming with the Western Interstate Commission for Higher Education Mental Health Program; Project management of a Department of Defense study on mental health education within the National Guard, including adaptation of the Mental Health First Aid curriculum for use with the military and veteran population; and assisting with development and implementation of the White House PREVENTS Initiative focused on veteran suicide. She has briefed at numerous local, national and international conferences. Winkel holds a M.P.A. from the University of Illinois and a Systems Thinking Certificate from Cornell University. She was awarded the Adjutant General Medal by Major General Hugo E. Salazar for her efforts in implementing the Coalition and strengthening support for Arizona's military, veteran and family population and recognized as one of the 48 Most Intriguing Women of Arizona as part of the state centennial.